KT-379-691

FAT AROUND THE MIDDLE

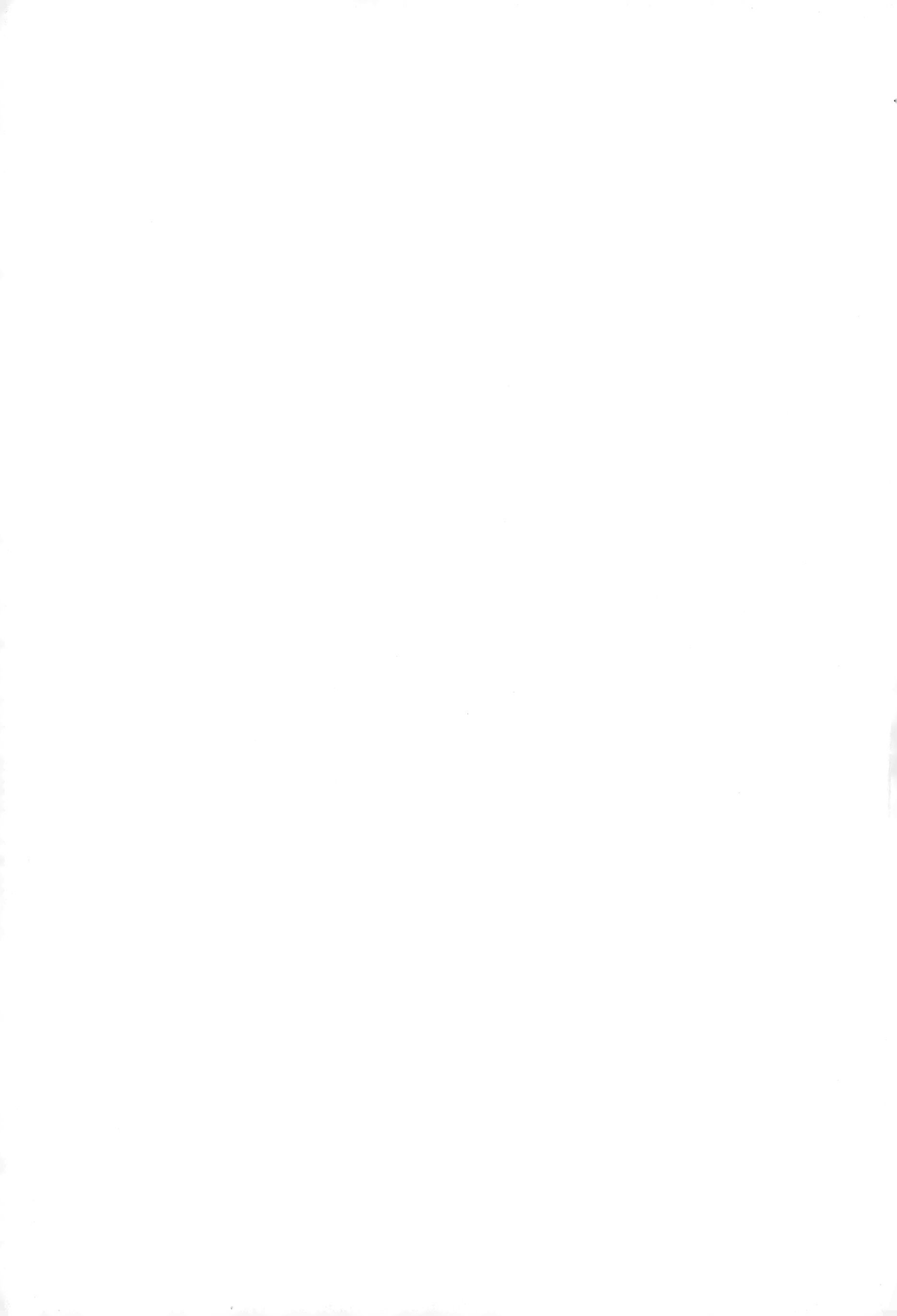

FAT AROUND THE MIDDLE

How to lose that bulge – for good

Marilyn Glenville PhD

Kyle Cathie Ltd

ACKNOWLEDGEMENTS

It is always a pleasure to thank those who have helped, whether directly or indirectly, in getting a book published.

Once again, Louise Atkinson has helped make me stay on track and not get so bogged down in the science that the message gets lost. My thanks also to Jenny Wheatley, my editor at Kyle Cathie, and to all the staff at Kyle Cathie for their professionalism and enthusiasm for this book.

Special thanks must go to all the team at the Tunbridge Wells clinic who work so efficiently and with a wonderful sense of humour to make sure everything continues to run smoothly. It is a privilege to thank Alison, Mel, Helen, Brenda, Jenny, Trine, Wendy, Nick and Sally for always working hard and with a passionate belief that what we do fundamentally makes a difference in people's lives, be it helping them to have a baby, getting through the menopause without drugs or losing that belly and staying healthy.

My love to all my family – to my husband Kriss for running the business side of the clinics, to free me up to do what I do best and to my children (now adults) Matt, Len and Chantell for just being who they are.

Disclaimer

The contents of this book are for information only and are intended to assist readers in identifying symptoms and conditions they may be experiencing. This book is not intended to be a substitute for taking proper medical advice and should not be relied upon in this way. Always consult a qualified doctor or health practitioner. The author and publisher cannot accept responsibility for illness arising out of the failure to seek medical advice from a doctor.

First published in Great Britain in 2006 by
Kyle Cathie Limited
122 Arlington Road, London NW1 7HP
general.enquiries@kyle-cathie.com
www.kylecathie.com

10 9 8 7 6

ISBN 1 85626 655 9
ISBN (13-digit) 978 1 85626 655 0

All rights reserved. No reproduction, copy or transmission of this publication may be made without written permission. No paragraph of this publication may be reproduced, copied or transmitted save with written permission or in accordance with the provision of the Copyright Act 1956 (as amended). Any person who does any unauthorised act in relation to this publication may be liable to criminal prosecution and civil claims for damages.

Marilyn Glenville is hereby identified as the author of this work in accordance with Section 77 of the Copyright, Designs and Patents Act 1988.

Text © 2006 Marilyn Glenville
Book design © 2006 Kyle Cathie Limited

Project editor: Jennifer Wheatley
Designer: Robert Updegraff
Illustrations pp166–175: Jennifer Wheatley
Copy editor: Anne Newman
Editorial assistant: Vicki Murrell
Production: Sha Huxtable and Alice Holloway

A Cataloguing In Publication record for this title is available from the British Library.

Printed and bound by Martins the Printers Ltd, Berwick upon Tweed

To Matt and Hannah –
may all your dreams come true

Marilyn Glenville PhD is the UK's leading expert in nutritional health for women. She obtained her doctorate from Cambridge University and is a Fellow of the Royal Society of Medicine as well as the Royal Society of Arts and is a member of the Nutrition Society.

For over twenty-five years Dr Glenville has studied and practised nutrition, both in the UK and in the US. She has had several papers published in scientific journals, frequently advises health professionals and often lectures at academic conferences held at the Medical Society, the Royal College of Physicians and the Royal College of Surgeons. She is also a popular international speaker. As a respected author on women's healthcare she gives regular talks on radio and has often appeared on television and in the press.

Dr Glenville is the editorial representative on the Forum for Food and Health at the Royal Society of Medicine and is also on the Medical Advisory Panel for the registered charity, Women's Health. She is patron of the Daisy Network, a premature menopause support group. Dr Glenville was formerly an observer on the Foods Standards Agency's Expert Group on the safety of vitamins and minerals.

She is also the author of several internationally best-selling books on health including: *Natural Alternatives to Dieting, The New Natural Alternatives to HRT, Healthy Eating for the Menopause, Osteoporosis, Natural Solutions to Infertility, The Nutritional Health Handbook for Women* and *Overcoming PMS the Natural Way*.

Dr Glenville runs her own clinics in London and Tunbridge Wells and also has a website: www.marilynglenville.com

CONTENTS

• **Introduction** •

Welcome to the Fat Around the Middle Plan

Are you frustrated with your body shape? Do you feel that your arms and legs look all right, yet the area from your bust to your groin seems to defy all your attempts to shrink it? Does it seem as though every sneaked chocolate biscuit or handful of crisps settles as fat around your middle? Do your clothes feel uncomfortable – maybe your skirts are too tight, your blouse gapes and a 'muffin top' layer of fat pours over the waistband of your jeans? Worst of all, have you been asked when your baby is due?

If so, this is the book for you. Its aim is to help you – and countless other women like you – to change your body shape for good.

Of course, your appearance is important, affecting, as it does, your confidence, self-esteem and self-image. However, the fat around your middle can also be dangerous. Scientists now know that storing fat in the middle of your body rather than anywhere else has major health implications and studies show that it increases the risk of heart disease, diabetes, stroke, cancer and high blood pressure.

So, appearances aside, it has never been more important that you do something about your body shape. The fact that you're reading this is a very good sign – it means that you are motivated and ready to set changes in motion. And the great benefit of following the recommendations in this book is that you will not only get rid of that fat around your middle – in as little as three months – but you will also be helping to prevent health problems in the future. So, in the short term, you get to look (and, therefore, feel) better. And in the long term? You live longer – it's as simple as that.

You don't have to be overweight to have fat around your middle. Even a lean woman of normal weight can have too much in the centre of her body and this still carries risks (see pictures opposite).

The reason why some people store fat around their middle whilst others do not has much to do with the way in which the body works. Every time you eat, your body will either burn your food as energy or store it as fat. In your case, and that of thousands like you, your body chooses to store your food as fat and also to store it in one particular place in your body.

Fat distribution

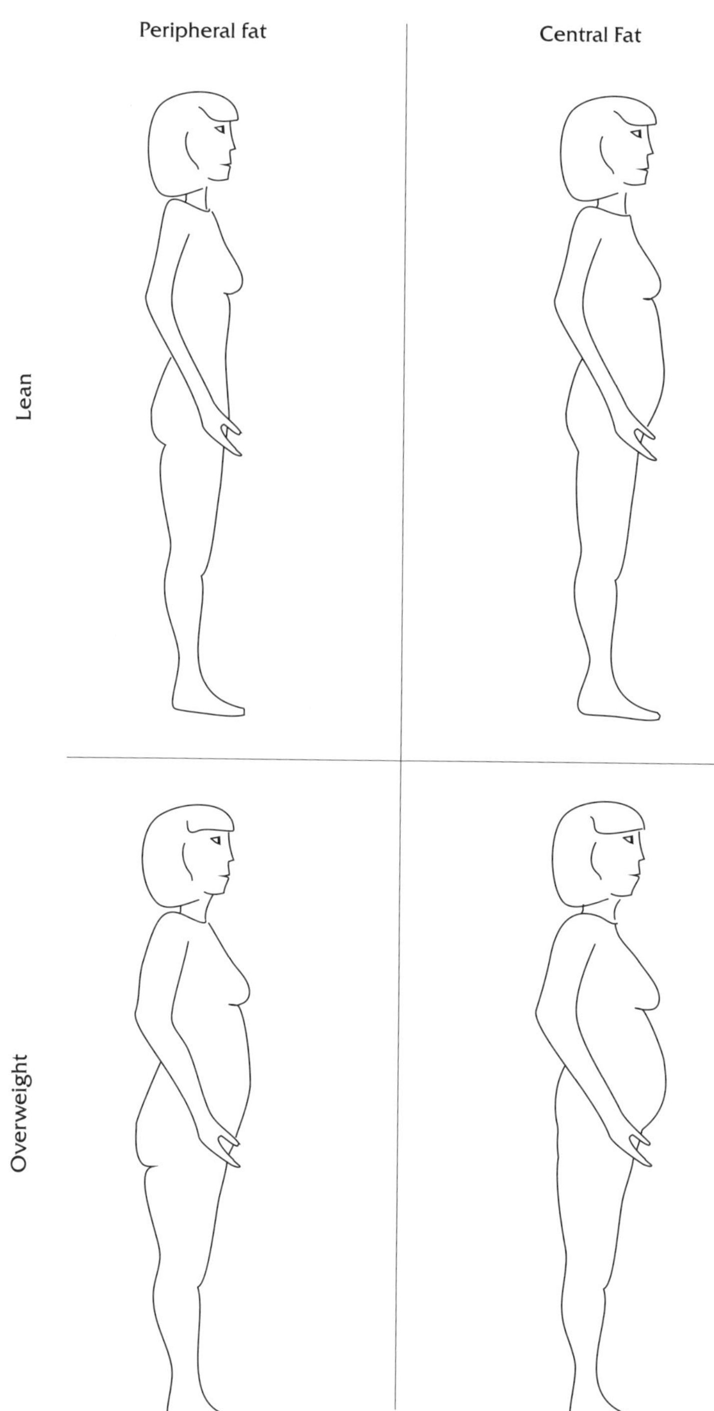

It is important, therefore, to realise that if your weight is sitting around the middle of your body, it is an indication of an imbalanced metabolism. This is something that needs to be addressed, and not simply by undertaking a weight-loss diet. So, rest assured, this is not just another diet book and food is not your main problem. Yes, of course, what you eat is important and the role of food and nutrition will be explained fully in Chapter 4. However, the aim here is to change your body's underlying biochemistry and let it know that it is all right for it to let go of the fat around the middle of your body.

As you start making the small changes recommended in this book you will begin to see your body changing shape and, at the same time, you will start to feel so much healthier. You'll have more energy, your mood will pick up, headaches will disappear and your skin and hair will also improve. All this will spur you on to go further and make more changes, taking you from a negative cycle into a positive one. And, for added motivation, you can now get a picture of yourself showing you what you might look like without that fat around the middle (see 'Slimmer You' photograph in the Resources section, page 183).

To get the most out of this book you should first read through chapters 1 to 9. This will give you a really good understanding of why your body is storing fat around the middle and the messages it has been receiving over the years to make that happen. Once you have done that, you will be ready for Chapter 10, 'Plan of Action', which takes you, step by step, through all the changes you should make and how to implement them. (Of course, you can go straight to Chapter 10 if you want to get stuck in straight away.) Follow up with Chapter 11 which gives recommendations for helping you to stay slim long term.

Although the plan is not a 'for ever' regime, most of the women who come to my clinic say that because they feel so much better and friends remark on how well they are looking, they continue to follow its recommendations most of the time.

We only get one body and, having worked in the healthcare service for twenty-five years, I have never been more certain that nothing is more important than good health. The choice is yours. Nobody else can take responsibility for your own health but you. So why not get started now, and within just three months you will have completely changed your body shape. You'll be back in clothes you thought you'd never be able to wear again and you will have got your energy back. And don't forget the added bonus – you will also have reduced your risk of life-threatening illnesses.

• Chapter 1 •

Why Your Body Stores Fat on the Waist

(And other women's bodies don't)

How You Respond to Stress

Shifting the fat around your middle has far less to do with your diet or lack of motivation in the aerobics class and much, much more to do with the action of stress hormones in your body. The main reason why some people gather more fat around their middle than others is very specifically because of the action of the stress hormone cortisol.

Fight or flight

Millions of years ago, our bodies were designed to react quickly to danger, just like wild animals, on constant alert to fight or run if threatened. Known as the 'fight-or-flight response', this is crucial for the survival of all animals – including humans. When your brain thinks that your life is under threat, it releases a substance called corticotrophin-releasing-hormone (CRH) which immediately stimulates the adrenal glands to release the hormones adrenaline and cortisol. At this point a number of physical changes take place in your body and these are dealt with in detail on page 13.

The fight-or-flight response is incredibly clever and thoroughly efficient, providing everything your body needs to react swiftly in dangerous situations. Once the threat is out of the way (you've either won the battle or escaped the attacker), the adrenal glands stop pumping out hormones and your body returns to normal.

The only problem is that evolution is lagging a little behind modern-day life. These days, many of us live under chronic stress but this stress comes from deadlines, traffic jams or children having tantrums, rather than from spear-wielding attackers or sabre-tooth tigers. The body can't distinguish between late trains, missed appointments, spiralling debt, family disputes and the truly life-threatening stress that it is geared up to challenge. So it reacts in exactly the same as way as it has always done – fight or flight.

Because stress as we know it today is almost continuous and comes without the natural release that either fighting or fleeing might provide, its effect on the body can be extreme, given that reactions designed to last for a five- to ten-minute period are operating for hours on end.

In a stressful situation, the adrenaline that is released helps to get you alert and focused, whilst the cortisol increases levels of fat and sugar in the bloodstream. However, unless you do something physical (as your body is expecting you to) all that extra energy, in the form of fat and glucose, has nowhere to go and must simply be re-deposited as fat.

After a stressful event, adrenaline levels will quickly return to normal and the body should be restored to a state of calm. But the level of cortisol often remains higher for a while (sometimes for as long as a few days), and because it thinks you should refuel your body after all this fighting or fleeing it increases your appetite. This is perfectly acceptable when you have been fighting or running for your life as your body will clearly need to stock up again. If, however, you've been chained to a desk fielding stressful phone calls, constant refuelling is hardly appropriate.

So, the bottom line here is that people under constant stress quite often feel hungry all the time. And worse still, their body urges them to stock up on the foods it thinks will be most useful after all that 'activity', namely carbohydrates and fats. If you indulge this, you'll inevitably gain weight.

The reason why I bring in the fight-or-flight mechanism so early in this book is because it is absolutely crucial. It is now widely accepted there is a strong connection between stress hormones and the formation of fat around your middle. If you don't fight or flee when your body expects you to, the fat and glucose swimming in your system will be deposited as fat around your middle. And any weight gain from anything sugary or fatty that you eat as a consequence of the post-stress appetite surge will also end up in the same place.

There is nothing random in this fat allocation. The reason why fat targets your middle is because it is close to the liver where it can most quickly be converted back into energy if needed. It provides you with a cunning (but infuriating) form of protection, ready for the next stress attack.

The General Adaptation Syndrome (GAS)

Stress specialists refer to the way in which the body reacts under pressure as the General Adaptation Syndrome (or GAS). Although I have already discussed the fight-or-flight response above, it is worth looking at it in slightly more detail because understanding GAS is the first step to implementing some changes in your life that will make fat around the middle less inevitable than you might think.

In the 1920s a medical student named Hans Selye identified the fact that all animals, from mice to humans, go through the same stages of stress:

Stage 1 – alarm

This is the fight-or-flight bit. It is usually short-lived but it is intense as your body goes on full alert:

- Your heart speeds up and your blood pressure rises.
- The clotting ability of your blood increases so that you will recover more quickly if you are injured and start to bleed.
- Your digestion shuts down (there's no need for it – you are unlikely to stop off for a quick sandwich if your life is in danger) and the energy needed for that system is diverted elsewhere.
- Your liver immediately releases emergency stores of glucose into the bloodstream to provide instant energy to fight or run.
- Your immune system produces more white blood cells so that you'll be better equipped to fight foreign viruses or bacteria.
- Your muscles tense and blood is moved away from the skin and internal organs (except the heart and lungs) and towards the muscles.
- Breathing becomes faster and shallower to supply oxygen to your brain, heart and muscles.
- Sweating increases to eliminate toxins produced by the body.
- Bladder and rectum muscles relax (in cases of extreme stress, you can either wet yourself or open your bowels, and many people get diarrhoea before an exam or job interview).
- Adrenaline is released directly into the bloodstream and cortisol levels rise, boosting blood sugar to give you energy. This is the stage at which the body is so pumped up that people have been known to do almost super-human feats, such as lifting up a car to free a trapped person underneath.

Once the first stage is over, the body should recover. Adrenaline levels come down fairly quickly and cortisol more slowly (days rather than hours). However, if the cause of stress is not removed, as so often happens in modern-day life, the body proceeds to stage 2.

Stage 2 – resistance

Cortisol maintains the fight-or-flight response by increasing blood sugar levels to keep energy going and by retaining sodium to keep blood pressure up. It also helps to stimulate the conversion of proteins, fats and carbohydrates into energy to help you in your ongoing 'battle'. Cortisol levels can remain high like this for a very long time, and in many cases the body seems to adapt to this constant level of stress. This is what really causes the fat around the middle. To continue providing the energy it thinks you need, the body needs to keep a convenient fat store ready for constant use. It also creates cravings and increases appetite to ensure good supplies of necessary fuel.

YOUR ADRENALS

To understand fully why your body puts fat around your middle when stress hormones are released, it is important to know what the adrenal glands actually do.

Cortisol and adrenaline are the two main stress hormones. They are produced by the adrenals which are two small glands located above the kidneys. The adrenal glands have been ideally placed in the body by Nature as they are only a short distance from the major artery of the body, the aorta, and also close to the major vein, the vena cava. This means that in times of stress, the hormone messages can be pumped into the bloodstream and transported very quickly to the rest of the body. The adrenals are also close to the liver and pancreas so that these organs can respond quickly (when triggered by cortisol) and can provide instant energy by pumping out stored glucose when needed.

Each adrenal gland is made up of two separate sections – the cortex and medulla.

The cortex

This is the larger, outer portion of the gland (making up 80–90 per cent of its bulk). It secretes three types of steroid hormone called corticosteroids. They are:

Glucocorticoids

The most significant glucocorticoid is cortisol which helps to regulate glucose metabolism. Cortisol also helps to control the metabolism of fat, protein and carbohydrate metabolism which means it has an impact on the production of energy, thyroid hormones and also on the immune system. Cortisol is released into the bloodstream at varying levels throughout the day, and the rhythm and timing of this is as important as the amount produced. It should be highest in the morning (when you are ready for the day ahead) and lowest at night (when you're going to bed).

Mineral corticoids

The most important mineral corticoid is aldosterone which controls salt and water balance in the body. It helps to regulate the reabsorption of sodium and the excretion of potassium by the kidneys. It is also one of the many hormones that can influence the development of high blood pressure.

DHEA

DHEA, otherwise catchily known as dehydroepiandrosterone, is the starting block for the sex hormones: oestrogen and testosterone. It also works on your behalf to reverse the effects of high cortisol levels, but at times when cortisol levels remain high (if you're under chronic stress), natural levels of DHEA will drop. DHEA is important for energy, sleep, preventing PMS, and sex drive.

The medulla

This is the smaller, inner portion of the adrenal glands and is made up of a mass of nerve tissue that secretes hormones called catecholamines which consist of adrenaline and noradrenaline.

Adrenaline

Known as epinephrine in the USA, this is the classic fight-or-flight hormone which triggers expansion of blood vessels, increased blood pressure, higher blood glucose levels and increased heart rate.

Noradrenaline

This hormone (known as norepinephrine in the USA) behaves in the opposite way to adrenaline, causing the blood vessels to constrict.

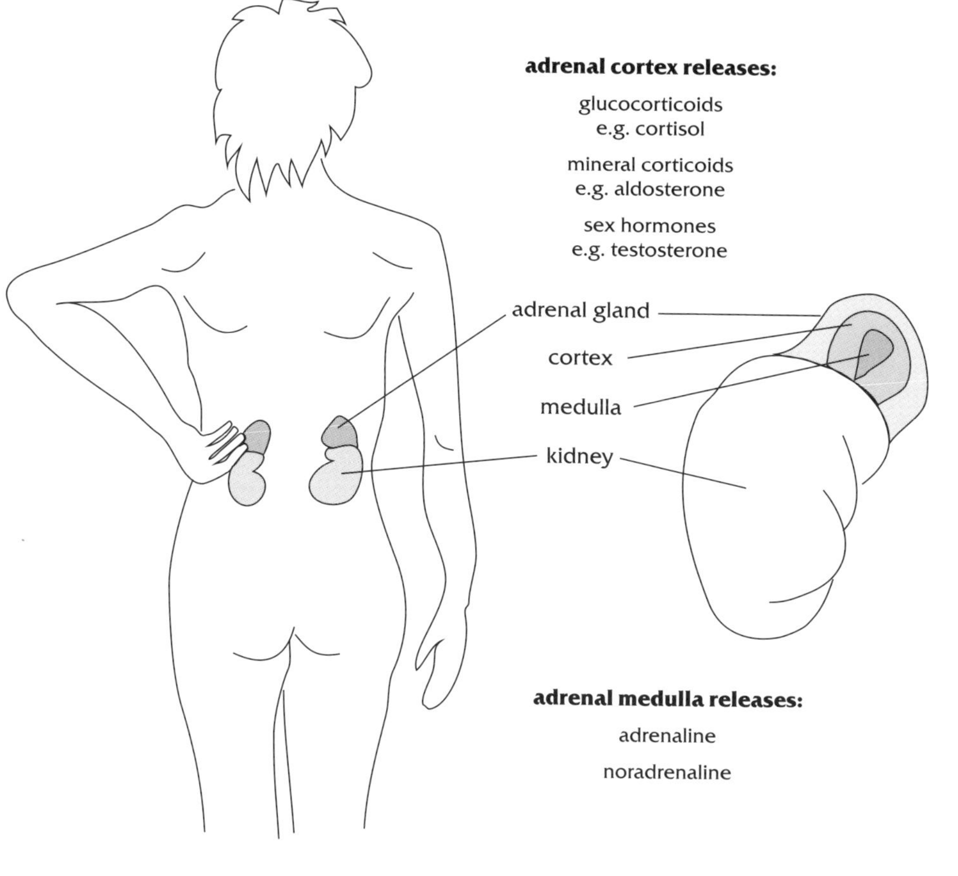

But in many, many people, stress is continuous and the body never gets the long periods of recovery it really needs. It's like driving a car with your foot on the accelerator the whole time – even when stationary – because fear and anxiety frequently continue even after a stressful situation has passed.

And there is only so long that the body can continue like this until it hits stage 3.

Stage 3 – exhaustion

This is when your body reaches the end of the line. It is close to a state of total collapse because the body just cannot keep functioning on overdrive. Cortisol levels drop dramatically as the adrenal glands finally give up their fight, and low blood sugar levels follow. The effect is a dramatic drop in energy levels which can be really quite debilitating.

Overcoming resistance

It is now extremely common to spend many years in resistance (stage 2) and, if you are accumulating fat around the middle of your body, the chances are that you are in this stage. Your body is simply doing the best it can to equip you for a constant onslaught of stress, to help you cope with the threats and anxieties it perceives you to be facing each day, and to keep you functioning as efficiently as possible.

Some people live their whole lives – seemingly quite happily – in resistance. They appear to recover after each setback and to continue 'living on adrenaline'. But their bodies are suffering, and they are very vulnerable. A major trauma, accident or bereavement could easily precipitate a complete collapse. Something relatively small can also be the last straw that tips a person over the edge. You may also know of people whose hair falls out (or turns white) after one shocking event and the body never fully recovers afterwards.

This is often known as a 'physical breakdown'. There are many examples. I treated a man who worked in the city, had a stressful job and (like so many) was burning the candle at both ends. He thought nothing of saying yes to a weekend rugby match, followed by a beery night with his friends, even though he was fighting a cold. It was, however, clearly too much for his poor, chronically stressed body. He collapsed in the pub and was rushed to hospital with an auto-immune condition which left him completely paralysed for days, and partially paralysed for months. He is now back at work, but, even a year on, one side of his face is still 'lazy' and will drop if he's tired.

Dr Selye, known as 'the grandfather of stress', and author of *The Stress of Life,*[1] said: 'No one can live without experiencing some degree of stress all the time. You may think that only serious disease or intensive physical or mental injury can cause stress. This is false. Crossing a busy intersection, exposure to a draught, or even sheer joy are enough to activate the body's stress mechanisms to some extent. Stress is not even necessarily bad for you; it is also the spice of life, for any emotion, any activity causes stress. But, of course, your system must be prepared to take it. The same stress which makes one person sick can be an invigorating experience for another.'

So, one thing that is absolutely clear from the research into how stress affects the body is that we all react to stress in different ways. Two apparently similar people can find themselves in exactly the same situation and one might find it extremely stressful whilst the other finds it wildly exciting. Take rollercoaster rides as an example – some people love them, others hate them. The ride is the same but each person's perception of it makes their experience different.

Stress makes some people want to eat more, whilst others will eat very little. Some people lose their appetite and even lose weight under stress, whilst others gain it at an alarming rate. And this is crucially important for this book. The key factor in terms of weight control is to think about how *your* body reacts to and copes with stress.

In one study, researchers gave puzzles to stimulate stress to a group of women then compared the results in those with a high waist-to-hip ratio (see page 27) to those of women with a low waist-to-hip ratio. They found that women with fat around the middle tended to produce more cortisol under stress and also reported having more stressful lives.[2]

Adrenal Disorders

Addison's disease and Cushing's syndrome are the two main adrenal disorders and each of them is caused by an extreme in the malfunctioning of the adrenal glands.

Addison's disease is a problem of hypofunction, meaning that the adrenal glands are simply not producing enough hormones. Symptoms can include weight loss, muscle weakness, fatigue, low blood pressure, hyperpigmentation (darkening of the skin), nausea, diarrhoea, dizziness, mood swings, lethargy and depression.

Cushing's syndrome is the result of the opposite extreme, where the adrenal glands are in a state of hyperfunction and are producing too many hormones. Symptoms include weight gain around the middle of the body, depression, insomnia, lack of sex drive, high blood pressure, insulin resistance, diabetes and, in women, irregular periods. Many of these symptoms are similar to the body's response to the extra cortisol released when you are under stress. Full-blown Cushing's syndrome is fairly rare but it does illustrate the subtle changes in your body shape and health that can take place through having just a few too many stress hormones floating around.

CORTISOL – THE DEVIL IN DISGUISE

It is quite clear that cortisol is responsible for telling your body to store fat, for increasing your appetite and for locking fat around your middle.[3] But cortisol is nevertheless an important hormone for the body so, as always, it is a question of balance.

Cortisol levels only rise too high (and stay raised) if your life is one of ongoing stress. High levels of the hormone mean that your body will think it needs to be continuously refuelling and storing fat around your middle ready to be called upon for energy to fight more stress. Under constant stress, the high cortisol level signals the liver to release its stores of glucose (fuel for energy) to cope with imminent 'attack'. Cortisol also tells the fat cells around the middle of your body to release fat for fuel – straight into the bloodstream. The result is that glucose (sugar) and fat are released ready for fight or flight, but if you remain seated at your desk or behind your steering wheel, silently fuming, the fat and sugar are not used up.

After a while, the high levels of blood sugar will trigger the pancreas to release the hormone insulin. This tells your body to store fat and triggers a craving for something sweet and fatty like chocolate. So rest assured it is not just weakness that draws you towards the fridge – it is an unassailable physical urge!

Unfortunately, abdominal fat cells have many receptors for cortisol (four times more than anywhere else in your body), so if you're too stressed and have high levels of cortisol, your abdominal fat cells will be calling out for it, encouraging your body to store more fat there. Which explains why fat accumulates so readily in that part of the body.

THE SYMPTOMS OF STRESS

Whatever the cause of your stress, if you are under pressure and your cortisol levels are high, you could be experiencing any of the following:

- a tendency to gain fat around your middle
- an increased appetite
- increased cravings for chocolate, sweets, breads, cakes, caffeine and alcohol (particularly any combination of carbohydrates and fats, such as chocolate and cakes because they are particularly high in calories)
- a slump in the middle of the afternoon, around three or four o'clock, when you know you are going to need a cup of tea or coffee and/or something sweet to get you through the afternoon
- a low immune system (you get frequent colds and infections)
- headaches
- nail biting or skin picking around the nails

WOMEN AND STRESS

Unfortunately, women are much more susceptible than men to the effects of stress, especially mental stress. We tend to worry more and have less of a laid-back attitude to life. I have seen women in the clinic who freely admit that they can 'worry for England'. So many women seem to have a natural urge to want to fix things and keep everybody happy. We are always thinking of other people, especially in the family, and trying to be all things to everyone. This is, obviously, very difficult to achieve – virtually impossible, in fact – and very stressful too.

Even though you may think you are not stressed – perhaps you've cut back on that high-pressure job to be with the children, or your debts are finally under some sort of control – you could be suffering from what has been dubbed the 'Hurried Woman Syndrome'. An American researcher called Dr Brent Bost has identified this as something experienced by women between the ages of twenty-five and fifty-five who are trying to do too many things in a short space of time. Typically, he says, they are rushed off their feet, juggling the demands of work, family life, household chores and caring for elderly relatives. In short, never-ending, ongoing stress.

Some women will have been exposed to many stressful life situations while others may be more vulnerable psychologically to stress, making them overreact to perceived stress. The end result is the same. Both groups of women will have had a greater lifetime exposure to cortisol.

- teeth grinding (the best way to tell if you are grinding is to attempt a bowl of muesli for breakfast – if your aching jaws steer you towards porridge, see your dentist about a cushioning bite guard)
- high cholesterol
- blood sugar swings
- digestive problems (such as bloating and flatulence)
- chest pains (you must see your doctor if you are getting chest pains, but the effects of the stress hormones can mimic heart problems)
- muscle aches and pains
- shoulder and neck pain (stress hormones will keep certain muscles tense ready for fight or flight)
- hair loss
- irregular or absent periods (your reproductive system is the only system your body can shut down without killing you, so when you are stressed your body may divert energy and resources away from your reproductive organs)
- difficulty in concentrating or forgetfulness
- depression

- increased premenstrual symptoms (PMS)
- a slower metabolism (which makes it harder to lose weight in general)
- a low sex drive
- tiredness, yet an inability to sleep well
- a tendency to get a second wind in the evening and/or waking up in the middle of the night, finding it hard to get back to sleep and then desperately wanting to sleep on in the morning when you should be getting up (these two are caused by your daily cortisol rhythm being out of sync – cortisol should be starting to rise in the morning ready for you to wake up and be alert and then quieten down at night ready for sleep)

TEST YOUR STRESS

How do you know if you are under stress? Most of us think we have a pretty good idea, but the important distinction is the degree to which stress is affecting your health. There are a number of ways of assessing stress (a laboratory test is discussed in Chapter 9) and a simple checklist (see opposite) can be a good start.

Psychologists have traditionally used something called the Social Readjustment Rating Scale. This was originally designed as a predictive tool to assess the likelihood of somebody falling victim to stress-related problems such as anxiety or depression. But it can also be used to give an indication of your level of stress.

Total up your scores for events that have happened to you over the past year from the list on the facing page. If a particular event has happened more than once within the last twelve months, multiply its value by the number of occurrences.

It might seem strange to include Christmas as it is an inevitable annual event, but the object of this checklist is to give you a good picture of how your stressful events add up over a full year. A lot of women find Christmas very stressful; what with buying presents, food shopping and preparation and then dealing with in-laws and other relatives, it can be the last straw in an already stressful year. Holidays are also listed as a stress event even though we go on holiday to relax. This is because many people find the lead-up to a holiday – preparing, packing, tying up loose ends – very stressful. And some families find that spending seven or fourteen days together away from home can also induce stress.

If you scored between 0 and 149 you have experienced a fairly low level of stressful events over the last year and psychologists would estimate that you have a 30 per cent chance of developing a stress-related illness or of becoming sick in the near future.

A score of between 150 and 299 gives you a 50 per cent chance of having a stress-related illness or of becoming unwell in the near future. You should take stock now and lower your stress levels in areas where you have some control.

Stress event	Score
Death of a spouse	100
Divorce	73
Marital (or other major intimate relationship) separation	65
Prison term	63
Death of a close family member	63
Personal injury or illness	53
Buying or moving house	50
Getting married	50
Being fired from work or made redundant	50
Caring for sick or elderly relative	47
Marital reconciliation	45
Change in health or behaviour of a family member	44
Pregnancy	40
Sexual difficulties	40
Gaining new family member through adoption or remarriage	39
Business changes	39
Change in financial state	38
Death of a close friend	37
Change of occupation	36
Increase in arguments with partner	35
Taking on a mortgage	35
Increase or decrease in responsibility at work	29
Son or daughter leaving home	29
Trouble with in-laws	29
Commuting	28
Spouse begins or stops work	26
Starting or leaving school/university	26
Change in living conditions	25
Change in personal habits	24
Trouble with boss	23
Change in working hours or conditions	20
Change in living conditions (e.g. building work)	20
Change in type and/or amount of recreation	19
Change in social activities	18
Major purchase (e.g. car)	17
Change in sleep quality	16
Change in number of family get-togethers	15
Holiday	13
Christmas	12
Minor violations of the law (e.g. speeding ticket)	11

Pay particular attention to your diet and see Chapter 5 for information on stress-busting supplements and herbs.

If you scored over 300 you have been through quite a year and it is really important that you start taking care of yourself now. From your score it would be estimated that there is an 80 per cent chance that you will become sick from a stress-related illness in the near future. You need to follow the recommendations in this book strictly to give your body and mind a chance to recover.

Whilst this type of questionnaire is useful it does not give you the total picture. The list above comprises what I call major stress events – clear-cut changes in your life. The kind of stresses that I come across most often in the clinic, however, and those that I would associate with fat around the middle are the stresses that affect us on a daily basis, putting us under constant pressure. It is the relentless round of chores and tasks that has to be completed in twenty-four hours, the juggling of all the balls just to get through the day. Take, for example, a working mother, whose early morning is in chaos as she gets the baby up, fed and dressed, dresses herself, then rushes to get to her train on time. She is stressed all day at work, then feels stressed and guilty for being a 'bad mother'. In the evenings and at weekends she catches up with cleaning and shopping and her daily life is spent trying to be a mother, partner, lover, daughter, work colleague, always with the constant feeling of 'no time for me'.

This is the kind of stress that eats away at you; it is there day in, day out, unlike the changes or 'stress events' in your life that are listed in the questionnaire above. Whilst these are undoubtedly stressful, they are a clear case of cause and effect. The daily stress, however, is unremitting with seemingly no way out because there is always so much to do, you are doing it all and everything depends on you. The result is that you end up with chronically elevated cortisol levels as your body thinks you are constantly fighting for your life, which, in a sense, you are.

You may find yourself resorting to a number of different coping patterns, including:

- overeating – especially sweet foods, chocolates, cakes, bread, etc.
- drinking too much alcohol
- using coffee and/or tea to get through the day
- overspending (using retail therapy as stress release)
- watching too much television (it stops you from thinking)
- smoking

You may also experience feelings of helplessness and wild mood swings – crying spells, aggression and anxiety.

FINDING A WAY FORWARD

You may find that you go to great lengths to relieve all this stress, making significant life changes, but that you still keep the fat around your middle. Why? This is because it takes time for your body to get the message that it is safe for it to let go of that weight and that the perceived threat is no longer there. Your body has been running in survival mode for so long that it will, for some time, continue to operate in that way.

That's the bad news.

The good news is that your body is very adaptable and once the weight does start to shift, your middle is the first place it comes off. Your body has to be given a new set of messages so that it can heal itself and learn to operate in a different way. Give yourself three months following the recommendations in this book and you will see the difference. Once you have got rid of that weight around your middle, you won't gain it back because when life seems to be getting too much or if you go through stress events you will see the signs quickly and know what to do.

• Chapter 2 •

GOOD OR BAD BODY FAT?

Why the fat around your middle won't disappear if you diet and how fat cells have a mind of their own

First of all, you should know that body fat is not all bad; everyone needs some body fat. It plays a critical role in various functions of the body, insulating us from the cold and keeping our skin and arteries supple. It also acts as a cushion, protects our organs and is an extremely handy source of stored energy. Too much, however, and in the wrong place, it can shorten your life.

• FAT CELL FACTS •

Fat cells begin forming whilst we are still in the womb and continue to form until we reach puberty. Women unfortunately have more fat cells than men. A man has 26 billion fat cells (or adipocytes), in his body whilst women, on average, have 35 billion. And a typical woman is made up of 27 per cent fat, yet men carry on average only 15 per cent of their body weight as fat. This is not a cruel trick of biology – it makes evolutionary sense. Fat is essential for reproduction to take place and Nature cunningly contrives to keep fat stored on the female body just in case a pregnancy occurs. Fat is also necessary for ovulation – if women lose too much body fat, their periods can stop. Again, Nature is no fool – if it registers a famine (low body fat) it figures food must be scarce so pregnancy might not be the best idea.

Once you reach puberty your designated supply of fat cells will have been allocated and however large or small that supply is the number of fat cells you carry around always remains the same. When you put on fat (your body siphons off excess food for storage purposes) you are not gaining new fat cells, merely 'filling' existing ones. No matter how much fat you gain you will not produce more fat cells, but your existing ones will swell up, sometimes as big as six times their minimum size. Conversely, when you lose weight the fat cells actually shrink.

Note: as with any rule there are always exceptions and it is possible for the body to create new fat cells during pregnancy (see page 31).

ARE YOU OVER-FAT OR OVERWEIGHT?

The most commonly accepted measure of whether or not someone is overweight is known as the Body Mass Index (BMI). This is the ratio of your height to your weight and is calculated by dividing your weight in kilograms by the square of your height in metres. For example, if your weight is 63.5kg (10 stone) and your height is 1.68m (5ft 6in), your BMI will be 63.5 ÷ 1.68 x 1.68 = 22.5 (see chart on page 26). This result of this calculation (usually a figure between 20 and 40) puts you, broadly speaking, into a weight category.

What does your BMI mean?

Under 20	underweight
20–25	normal
25–30	overweight
30–40	obese
Over 40	dangerously obese

It is startling to learn that the average BMI in the UK today stands at 24.5 – right at the top of the 'normal' rating and rather too close to 'overweight'. There is little doubt that the UK is on the verge of an obesity epidemic and it is estimated that one in three adults will be dangerously overweight within fifteen years if fundamental changes to diet and lifestyle are not made.

Obesity causes at least 30,000 deaths a year in the UK, from medical conditions such as heart disease, stroke and diabetes. With a BMI of just 25 (that's 60 per cent of UK women and 70 per cent of men) your risk of diabetes is five times greater than that of someone with a BMI of 22; if your BMI is 30 (20 per cent of women in the UK and 22 per cent of men) your risk is twenty-eight times greater.[1] It's a sobering thought and one that reinforces the fact that being overweight is clearly bad for you.

The drawback of the BMI as a measure, however, is that it cannot allow for variations in fat, bone, organs and muscle. Muscle tends to be heavier than fat, so the BMI of a 'well-built', extremely fit person might be as high as that of an unfit, rather fat person. Similarly, it is quite feasible to be over-fat and yet not overweight, and to register, therefore, a relatively low BMI. That does not mean you're safe and healthy, however. It is extremely important to consider where your fat is situated.

So how can you measure your body fat? Until relatively recently, gyms would attack their clients with giant pincers, so that they could literally 'pinch an inch' of fat at various points around the body and so calculate (roughly) how much fat there was. Today fat percentage machines can be found at every gym or purchased for the price of a good set of bathroom scales. You either grip each side of a machine with both hands, or stand on a modified set of scales

USE THIS CHART TO FIND YOUR BODY MASS INDEX

Imperial measures given are only approximates.

Height in centimetres

Weight in kilograms	142	145	147	150	152	155	158	160	163	165	168	170	173	175	178	180	183	Weight in stones and pounds
40	20	19	19	18	17	17	16	16	15	15	14	14	13	13	13	12	12	**6st 4**
41	20	20	19	18	18	17	16	16	15	15	15	14	14	13	13	13	12	**6st 6**
42	21	20	19	19	18	17	17	16	16	15	15	15	14	14	13	13	13	**6st 9**
43	21	20	20	19	19	18	17	17	16	16	15	15	14	14	14	13	13	**6st 11**
44	22	21	20	20	19	18	18	17	17	16	16	15	15	14	14	14	13	**6st 13**
45	22	21	21	20	19	19	18	18	17	17	16	16	15	15	14	14	13	**7st 1**
46	23	22	21	20	20	19	18	18	17	17	16	16	15	15	15	14	14	**7st 3**
47	23	22	22	21	20	20	19	18	18	17	17	16	16	15	15	15	14	**7st 6**
48	24	23	22	21	21	20	19	19	18	18	17	17	16	16	15	15	14	**7st 8**
49	24	23	23	22	21	20	20	19	18	18	17	17	16	16	15	15	15	**7st 10**
50	25	24	23	22	22	21	20	20	19	18	18	17	17	16	16	15	15	**7st 12**
51	25	24	24	23	22	21	20	20	19	19	18	18	17	17	16	16	15	**8st**
52	26	25	24	23	23	22	21	20	20	19	18	18	17	17	16	16	16	**8st 3**
53	26	25	25	24	23	22	21	21	20	19	19	18	18	17	17	16	16	**8st 5**
54	27	26	25	24	23	22	22	21	20	20	19	19	18	18	17	17	16	**8st 7**
55	27	26	25	24	24	23	22	21	21	20	19	19	18	18	17	17	16	**8st 9**
56	28	27	26	25	24	23	22	22	21	21	20	19	19	18	18	17	17	**8st 11**
57	28	27	26	25	25	24	23	22	21	21	20	20	19	19	18	18	17	**9st**
58	29	28	27	26	25	24	23	23	22	21	21	20	19	19	18	18	17	**9st 2**
59	29	28	27	26	26	25	24	23	22	22	21	20	20	19	19	18	18	**9st 4**
60	30	29	28	27	26	25	24	23	23	22	21	21	20	20	19	19	18	**9st 6**
61	30	29	28	27	26	25	24	24	23	22	22	21	20	20	19	19	18	**9st 9**
62	31	29	29	28	27	26	25	24	23	23	22	21	21	20	20	19	19	**9st 11**
63	31	30	29	28	27	26	25	25	24	23	22	22	21	21	20	19	19	**9st 13**
64	32	30	30	28	28	27	26	25	24	24	23	22	21	21	20	20	19	**10st 1**
65	32	31	30	29	28	27	26	25	24	24	23	22	22	21	21	20	19	**10st 3**
66	33	31	31	29	29	27	26	26	25	24	23	23	22	22	21	20	20	**10st 6**
67	33	32	31	30	29	28	27	26	25	25	24	23	22	22	21	21	20	**10st 8**
68	34	32	31	30	29	28	27	27	26	25	24	24	23	22	21	21	20	**10st 10**
69	34	33	32	31	30	29	28	27	26	25	24	24	23	23	22	21	21	**10st 12**
70	35	33	32	31	30	29	28	27	26	26	25	24	23	23	22	22	21	**11st**
71	35	34	33	32	31	30	28	28	27	26	25	25	24	23	22	22	21	**11st 3**
72	36	34	33	32	31	30	29	28	27	26	26	25	24	24	23	22	21	**11st 5**
73	36	35	34	32	32	30	29	29	27	27	26	25	24	24	23	23	22	**11st 7**
74	37	35	34	33	32	31	30	29	28	27	26	26	25	24	23	23	22	**11st 9**
75	37	36	35	33	32	31	30	29	28	28	27	26	25	24	24	23	22	**11st 11**
76	38	36	35	34	33	32	30	30	29	28	27	26	25	25	24	23	23	**12st**
77	38	37	36	34	33	32	31	30	29	28	27	27	26	25	24	24	23	**12st 2**
78	39	37	36	35	34	32	31	30	29	29	28	27	26	25	25	24	23	**12st 4**
79	39	38	37	35	34	33	32	31	30	29	28	27	26	26	25	24	24	**12st 6**
80	40	38	37	36	35	33	32	31	30	29	28	28	27	26	25	25	24	**12st 8**
81	40	39	37	36	35	34	32	32	30	30	29	28	27	26	26	25	24	**12st 11**
82	41	39	38	36	35	34	33	32	31	30	29	28	27	27	26	25	24	**12st 13**
83	41	39	38	37	36	35	33	32	31	30	29	29	28	27	26	26	25	**13st 1**
84	42	40	39	37	36	35	34	33	32	31	30	29	28	27	27	26	25	**13st 3**
85	42	40	39	38	37	35	34	33	32	31	30	29	28	28	27	26	25	**13st 5**
86	43	41	40	38	37	36	34	34	32	32	30	30	29	28	27	27	26	**13st 8**
87	43	41	40	39	38	36	35	34	33	32	31	30	29	28	27	27	26	**13st 10**
88	44	42	41	39	38	37	35	34	33	32	31	30	29	29	28	27	26	**13st 12**
89	44	42	41	40	39	37	36	35	33	33	32	31	30	29	28	27	27	**14st**
90	45	43	42	40	39	37	36	35	34	33	32	31	30	29	28	28	27	**14st 2**
	4ft 8	4ft 9	4ft 10	4ft 11	5ft 0	5ft 1	5ft 2	5ft 3	5ft 4	5ft 5	5ft 6	5ft 7	5ft 8	5ft 9	5ft 10	5ft 11	6ft	

Height in feet and inches

with bare feet. An electric current is passed (painlessly) though the body and the machine measures how long it takes for the current to go from one hand (or one foot) to the other. Lean tissue is a much better conductor of electricity than fatty tissue, so the more muscular you are, the quicker the current will pass. The more fat you have, the slower the current. The speed is then converted into a 'fat percentage' score. It is painless and pretty accurate.

How much is too much?

Individuals vary enormously and, as I mentioned earlier, women naturally carry more fat than men. Furthermore, we all tend to carry more fat as we get older as we become less active and lose muscle. Here's how the figures should look:

Healthy body fat

Age	Healthy percentage
18–29	19–24
30–39	20–26
40–59	21–28
60–79	22–29

However, I believe that the most important figure in determining your future health and well-being is neither your BMI, nor your body fat percentage score, but a far simpler measurement – the difference in size between your hips and your waist. This is the true measure of fat around the middle and the best indicator of whether or not you are going to be vulnerable to all the health risks associated with it.

If you have a spare tyre and can pinch a roll of fat around your middle you already know that you need to follow the recommendations in this book. But we all need a little 'flex', and we're not all built like supermodels. So how do you work out how much is too much?

Take a tape measure and compare your waist measurement (at the narrowest point) with your hip measurement (at the widest point). Divide the waist figure by the hip figure to get what is known as your waist-to-hip ratio.

For example, 86cm (34in) (waist) ÷ 94cm (37in) (hip) = 0.9.

A figure greater than 0.8 means that you are apple shaped and you need to keep reading; below 0.8 means that you are pear shaped and should pass this book on to a friend who might need it!

It is important to realise that any two women could be the same weight, have the same BMI and even the same fat percentage, yet if one of them carries her weight around her waist rather than her thighs and bottom she is at a much greater risk of suffering from serious illness.

The waist-to-hip ratio is an easy indicator of potential problems but one that is often overlooked by the medical profession. Our weight and height are usually measured during health checks but not our waist circumference. Why is it overlooked? One comment from a medical journal stated that 'many

BALLOONING WAISTLINES

Research from the Department of Health in 2005 shows that people in the UK now have the fattest stomachs recorded in history. Between 1993 and 2004, women's waistlines ballooned by an average of 4.1cm (1½in) to 86.6cm (34in), and men's by an average of 3.8cm (1½in) to 97.5cm (38½in). Figures published in 2004 showed that between 1951 and 2005, women's waists increased by 16.5cm (6½in).

But compare the other changes in height, bust and hips:

	1951	2004	Difference
Height	1.60m (5ft 3in)	1.63m (5ft 4½in)	3cm (1½in)
Bust	93cm (37in)	96cm (38½in)	3cm (1½in)
Hips	98cm (39in)	101cm (40½in)	3cm (1½in)
Waist	69cm (27½in)	85cm (34in)	16cm (6½in)

Source: National Sizing Survey

So we have become generally taller and larger but there is a huge difference between the 3cm (1½in) gains in height, bust and hips and the 16cm (6½in) gained on the waist. There is no doubt that we have lost the traditional hourglass figure (synonymous with a pear shape); women have become more apple shaped and therefore more vulnerable to the associated health risks.

physicians are more comfortable offering a plasma insulin level and prescribing insulin-sensitising medications than measuring a waist circumference and discussing diet and physical activity.'[2]

TUMMY FAT IS TOXIC FAT

Scientists always assumed that fat was just a useful form of energy storage. Getting enough to eat was the focus of survival and fat cells could be easily plundered in times of famine or attack. In the last few years, however, they have discovered that fat actually has a mind of its own, acting just like an endocrine (hormone-secreting) organ, producing its own array of hormones.[3]

Fat, also known as adipose tissue, manufactures an array of chemical messengers including blood-clotting agents, substances which contract blood vessels and raise blood pressure (vasoconstrictors), inflammatory agents, hormones and molecules which control hunger. Fat cells are also able to produce an immune response in the body, which causes inflammation. In evolutionary terms, this inflammatory response allowed the fat stores to help fight infection. Fat cells also secrete oestrogen and two other compounds – tumour necrosis factor alpha and resistin – both of which interfere with the functioning of insulin.

Unfortunately, not all fat in the body behaves in the same way and it is the fat around the middle of the body (or visceral fat, see box below) that has a mind of its own. This fat is far more metabolically active than fat elsewhere and has been called 'toxic fat' because it increases the risk of heart disease, high blood pressure, stroke, cancer and diabetes. The pear-shaped fat around the hips and thighs does not appear to operate in the same way and is relatively inactive and inert.

Fat cells around the waist have been found to be the most highly active of all. They pump out substances which might be quite useful in small doses, but when too much of this type of fat is active in this way the body's delicate balance can be upset. This can affect the way in which insulin is used and also raise blood pressure and increase the amount of cholesterol in the body. Abdominal fat cells can quickly break down stored fats, in case extra is needed when you are 'under attack' (see page 11). It then dumps the resulting fatty acids into the bloodstream which can cause high levels of fat and sugar in the blood. Whilst this may be useful if your life is in danger, when it is not (as is most often the case) it increases the risk of diabetes (in the case of blood sugar) and heart disease (in the case of fat).

• TYPES OF FAT CELL •

Subcutaneous or peripheral fat is stored beneath the skin and acts as an insulator to protect you against extremes of weather and to cushion your body so that you can sit comfortably in a chair. This kind of fat, which tends to sit around the hips and thighs, is relatively harmless.

Visceral or central fat serves as a shock absorber and protective shield to the vital organs of the body such as heart, liver, kidneys, brain and spinal cord. We all need some visceral fat to protect our organs but it is this central fat (some of which we can't see because it is deep inside our bodies) that can cause problems if there is too much of it. It is this kind of fat that makes up the apple shape.

The bodies of all children (girls and boys alike) start off straight up and down without a waist (small apple). Boys tend to stay that way as they grow into men, but when girls reach puberty they either stay apple shaped or become pear shaped and the way this goes seems to be largely genetically determined. Pear-shaped women appear to be driven more by the hormone oestrogen, which gives them a much more feminine, curvy, hourglass figure, usually associated with fertility and giving birth. Apple-shaped women have a more masculine form driven more by testosterone. This difference is not a problem in itself and only becomes sinister when the apple-shaped woman gains weight because she will inevitably gain visceral fat which then sits around the middle of her body carrying all the health risks I've discussed earlier.

CHUBBY TUMMY OR SYNDROME X?

There is a fine line between just having a chubby tummy and the point at which it causes health problems. Scientists studying the frightening preponderance of problems associated with apple-shaped fat distribution have given it a name: metabolic syndrome. It is also known as syndrome X or insulin resistance.

The big worry is that fat situated around the middle can kick off a domino effect which cascades all through the body, affecting many different areas. The problem we tend to think of as a cosmetic one can very rapidly snowball into wide-ranging and catastrophic problems such as heart disease, diabetes, stroke, high blood pressure and even cancer.

How does the domino effect start?

Cortisol has much to answer for. As we know, high cortisol levels mean high levels of blood sugar (glucose) because your body has to make sure that you have enough fuel to deal with imminent attack. When blood sugar increases, your body has to respond by releasing insulin from the pancreas to help move the glucose out of your blood and into the cells to provide them with energy. But if you don't need that energy (you don't fight or flee – see page 11) the default mechanism is to store the glucose as fat.

If the stress continues (and it usually does) cortisol levels remain high, so the body makes further attempts to increase blood sugar levels by triggering the breakdown of sugar stores in the liver and muscles. This is what gives you a craving for sugar or caffeine (as your body is urging you to refuel).

Out comes more insulin to deal with the extra blood glucose. And so it goes on… and that's all fine – for a while. The body is a well-oiled machine, adept at coping with blood sugar peaks and troughs. But over time, the body simply cannot respond to insulin in the same way it used to. If you push yourself to the limit too often you could easily become intolerant to insulin – or insulin resistant.

Insulin resistance

Insulin not only regulates your blood sugar but also fat storage. It ensures that sugar gets stored in our livers and muscle cells (in the form of glycogen) to help in muscle building. When you are under stress, cortisol tells the body not to store energy because it thinks you're going to need it for the fight-or-flight response. It's as if the cells get lazy, and stop responding to insulin. The fat cells dump more fat into the bloodstream, the liver cells produce more glucose and muscle cells allow their protein to be broken down to supply amino acids to be converted into more sugar by the liver.

Your body does a marvellous job of adapting to the situation up to a point, after which a whole host of problems can follow. Insulin resistance is the start of the problem and it is the hub of a wheel out of which radiate a number of frightening spokes (see page 37).

PLUMPING UP THE APPLE

Women of all ages can have fat around the middle for any of the reasons discussed in this book but there are some times in our lives when we are more likely to change shape than at others. These include pregnancy, after giving birth, whilst breastfeeding and in the menopause.

Pregnancy

Pregnancy is one of those times in our lives when the message to store fat is extremely powerful.

Women are also much more susceptible to blood sugar problems during pregnancy than they are at any other time in their lives. Gestational diabetes, for instance, can start during pregnancy and then (usually) disappears straight after the birth. Half of all women who have had gestational diabetes, however, are more likely to develop full-blown Type 2 diabetes within ten to fifteen years of giving birth.[4] Sufferers tend to gain weight during the pregnancy and normally give birth to much larger babies as their higher blood sugar levels cause the baby to grow more rapidly than otherwise.

Even in a healthy pregnancy, cortisol levels rise, peaking at the end of the third trimester[5], and with higher cortisol comes an increased susceptibility to blood sugar swings in pregnancy. Together with hormones produced during pregnancy these higher cortisol levels can work to block the action of insulin. This results in a tendency for most women to be insulin resistant during pregnancy and for a small percentage (up to 4 per cent) to end up with temporary (gestational) diabetes.

The fact that there is a higher risk of gestational diabetes in women over the age of thirty-five may help to explain why slightly older women tend to end up with more weight around the middle after a later pregnancy even if they don't develop gestational diabetes.

It has also been shown that women who have very high levels of cortisol during pregnancy have babies with high levels of cortisol which can remain for as long as ten years after the birth. This may manifest as psychological problems in the children and some experts think that prenatal stress should be thought of in the same way as smoking and alcohol in terms of negative effects on the baby.[6]

After birth and in the postnatal period, cortisol levels can still remain high in some women[7] making it more difficult to lose weight after the pregnancy. However, following the recommendations in this book strictly for three months should make it possible to get the body back into balance.

If you have had a baby and are thinking of having another it is important to get rid of the fat around your middle before going into the next pregnancy. There are two reasons for this. Firstly, it is never healthy to be pregnant and overweight, as this increases the risk of higher blood pressure and other problems like varicose veins. Secondly, if you start off a pregnancy with higher levels of insulin you can raise the risk of a number of problems including increased weight gain throughout the pregnancy, water retention and obesity postnatally and an increased risk of gestational and Type 2 diabetes in the future.[8]

Older pregnancies

If you had a baby in your late thirties or early forties you may find it even harder than others to shift the weight around your middle.

One reason for this is that although you may not notice it, your body is gearing up to prepare for menopause. It's not unusual to experience the odd hot flush when you're as young as thirty-five, or 'night sweats' if you are breastfeeding as your hormones rise and fall. Some women find that their periods don't restart once they stop breastfeeding or that they have a couple and then stop for good.

The reason for this apparently abrupt change is that your body goes through such an enormous hormonal upheaval during pregnancy. There is a huge surge in hormone levels for months followed by a massive drop after the birth. This is also a time of maximum fat storage as your body fights to hold on to any fat you gained during pregnancy so that it has enough reserves to help you feed the baby. You need 650 or so extra calories each day to produce breast milk. Also, during breastfeeding the hormone prolactin stays high to try to prevent you from ovulating and to protect you from getting pregnant again too soon. This means that the ovaries are almost 'dormant' during the whole period of the pregnancy and breastfeeding. In some women who are in their late thirties and early forties the ovaries don't 'kick-start' again once they stop breastfeeding and they actually go into early menopause.

If you are going into the menopause, your body will be extremely reluctant to let go of the fat around your middle. This is because fat is a manufacturing plant for oestrogen. Menopause happens because your natural oestrogen levels are falling and your body knows that any oestrogen your fat cells can produce will help to protect your bones from osteoporosis. It's a very clever system designed to protect you, but it does mean that mere diet and exercise alone will rarely shift that stubborn fat.

Pregnancy and birth are stressful events in themselves. The stress is even greater if you combine looking after a newborn with caring for other young children. The sheer physicality of the task gets tougher as you get older. Your body does not bounce back after the pregnancy quite as it would have done when you were younger and you don't have the same energy levels. You may find yourself snatching convenience and energy foods and drinks to give yourself a quick boost, or because you don't have the time or energy to feed yourself properly when you have other mouths to feed. It is all perfectly natural and understandable, but the message you will be unwittingly giving your body, loud and clear, is: 'This is a time of great stress; whatever you do, store fat!'

The menopause

As we grow older we tend to gain weight. We generally become less active, but we also naturally lose muscle and this makes it harder to burn fat. Whilst this is a problem experienced by men and women alike, women have the added complication of the hormonal changes of menopause.

The peri-menopause can start up to ten to fifteen years before the menopause. Many women will have no symptoms at all, except an expanding waistline and possibly their periods becoming more irregular as the function of the ovaries starts to decline. However, although we associate the menopause with the archetypal image of the 'matronly' woman with the large belly, it does not have to be that way.

The menopause creates something of a Catch-22 situation. As your ovaries produce less and less oestrogen, your body strives to compensate by manufacturing it elsewhere to protect your bones from osteoporosis. We know that larger and fatter women produce more oestrogen, which reduces their risk of osteoporosis, but the higher oestrogen levels do increase their risk of breast cancer.

It's a question of balance. The ultimate health goal is to have good enough levels of oestrogen to protect your bones without the levels increasing your risk of breast cancer.

For many women, the menopause itself is a source of stress. In our Western culture, it is seen as a negative state, a time of loss. No more periods mean you are no longer fertile (particularly poignant for women who could not have children). The chances are you'll also be experiencing the empty nest syndrome with children leaving home. You may be wondering what your role is now, or caring for sick elderly parents and wondering when it's all going to end. It all adds to the stress.

In more traditional cultures, the menopause is seen as a positive time, women gain status, they become 'wise women', extended families living together mean that they do not have to shoulder the entire responsibility of looking after elderly relatives and children do not move far away.

Unfortunately, cortisol, which as you know is produced when you are under stress, increases the activity of an enzyme called aromatase causing the body to convert more male hormones to oestrogen. This in turn causes the weight to pile on around the middle of your body[9] and therefore increases your risk of breast cancer.

So the combined effect of female hormonal changes, slower metabolism and stress with high cortisol levels come together to create a bigger likelihood of fat around the middle.

If you are approaching the menopause it is even more important for you to follow the recommendations in this book than anyone else, as you have to keep that shape change under control.

THE MEN IN YOUR LIFE

When men gain weight it is natural for them to gain it around the torso. And although men generally seem less bothered about being apple shaped, all the risks associated with having fat around the middle (heart disease, diabetes, high blood pressure, Alzheimer's, stroke and cancer) apply to men as well as women. In fact the risk of heart attack is much greater amongst men than it is in women.

There is no doubt that the weight around a man's middle increases his risk of a heart attack, in the same way that it does for women, because of the way in which the abdominal fat cells can quickly break down stored fats and dump the resulting fatty acids in the bloodstream. This can cause high levels of cholesterol, triglycerides (blood fats) and blood sugar. The body pumps out insulin to deal with the high blood sugar then, over time, the insulin becomes ineffective (insulin resistance, see page 30). This damages the arteries (atherosclerosis) causing debris (plaque) to fill and close them and in time this can lead to a heart attack. The narrowing of the arteries can also give rise to high blood pressure as the heart works harder and harder to pump the blood through ever-narrowing tubes. Sometimes as the debris piles up, a 'ball' of it can break away and trigger a clot which can result in either a heart attack or stroke.

Hormonal changes in men

As men get older they produce ever lower levels of testosterone. It's a gradual process, unlike the sudden change experienced by women at the menopause. However, this drop in testosterone has been called the 'male menopause' or 'andropause' where in some men the drop is severe enough to give them symptoms such as lack of sex drive, lethargy and lack of motivation.

As testosterone levels drop, muscle mass also shrinks which means that without regular exercise it will be harder to burn off fat (see Chapter 6). A natural slowing of the metabolism with age together with high levels of cortisol from stress can further decrease male hormone levels leading to weight piling on around the middle of the body. The obesity itself can cause male hormone levels to be 30–40 per cent lower than they are in slimmer men[10] and because lower levels of male hormones go hand in hand with reduced muscle mass, the overweight man will find it increasingly hard to lose weight and ever easier to put it on.

A man's fat is as much a manufacturing plant for oestrogen as a woman's which explains why men who have fat around the middle can end up with 'breasts'. The fat cells contain aromatase which, as we have seen, converts testosterone to oestrogen, so adding to the decline in testosterone for men, reducing their muscle mass and making it harder for them to lose weight.

Any man seeking to keep weight off his middle should take steps to reduce stress, increase exercise, improve diet and get enough sleep (this is crucial, as male hormones are released when sleeping). Alcohol is also an important factor for men. Not only does the alcohol supply carbohydrates in a liquid form (which means that they hit the bloodstream quickly, triggering high levels of insulin), but it also has a toxic effect on the testes, the organs which produce fat-busting testosterone.

If one of the men in your life looks worryingly large around the middle, take a tape measure to his tummy. If his waist-to-hip ratio (see page 27) is more than 0.95 he needs to take action now! It would also be worthwhile for him to do both the adrenal stress and the insulin resistance tests in Chapter 9 to see where he stands to begin with and then see the difference after three months of following the advice in this book.

• Chapter 3 •

How Your Fat Could Be Killing You

How the fat around your middle puts you at greater risk of breast cancer, heart disease and diabetes

If your body harbours fat around your middle, there is a strong chance that you are – to a greater or lesser extent – insulin resistant. This means that the constantly high levels of cortisol in your blood have confused your system. Your cells have been bombarded by insulin over such a long period of time that they no longer know what they're supposed to do. Significantly, they fail to do what insulin is telling them to do (i.e. to move glucose – blood sugar – into the cells) and so glucose levels remain high, and the high insulin tells your body to store fat.

This insulin resistance can trigger a host of other problems. Imagine a wheel with insulin resistance as the hub and all the other health problems radiating off from it on different spokes. Research has shown that the result of insulin resistance is like that of dropping a small pebble in a pond and watching the effect ripple across the water. So insulin resistance is connected with seemingly unrelated illnesses like cancer and Alzheimer's.

However, on the basis that insulin resistance lies at the core, if we eliminate that we can eliminate or at least reduce the risk of the diseases on the spokes of the wheel. The trick is to treat the cause, not the symptoms.

So how are all the diseases above connected to insulin resistance?

Heart Disease and Stroke

Normally when you eat, insulin tells the liver not to release fats into the bloodstream. This is important because your body is trying to deal with fat from the meal and does not want to deal with extra fat released from the liver. But when the liver is exposed to insulin for long periods of time (as a result of all your cortisol action), it starts to ignore the insulin and releases fats (as triglycerides) into the bloodstream. These fats are wrapped up in VLDLs (very low density lipoproteins) that are normally rendered harmless by enzymes in the blood. But because you are eating, these enzymes are otherwise occupied with dealing with the fat from your food. This means that the VLDLs are not

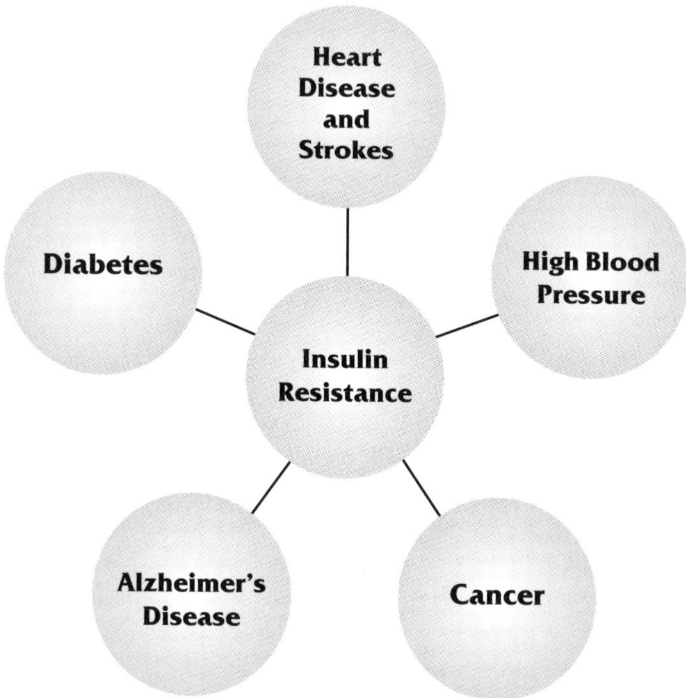

challenged and are free to stick to the walls of the arteries as plaque (an artery-clogging process called atherosclerosis).

In addition, less HDL is formed ('good' cholesterol which usually removes 'bad' cholesterol from the arteries), so the risk of heart disease is further increased because the cholesterol will build up in the blood vessels.

When you cut yourself, your body uses fibrinogen to help your blood to clot and prevent you from bleeding to death. In a fight-or-flight situation it is important to have this in the blood as your body must assume that you might get wounded. However, if the stress in question is a traffic jam or a looming deadline, the blood-clotting agent will be merely thickening your blood for no reason. This means that your arteries, already narrowed by fats, will be more susceptible to a spontaneous clot caused by high levels of fibrinogen. The end result could be a heart attack or stroke (if the clot is in the brain).

Of course, your body has a defence against this. It produces clever substances that dissolve clots once any repair process is under way. But the clot-removing process is hampered by a substance called PAI-1 (plasminogen activator inhibitor-1) which the high cortisol levels ensure is high in the blood at times of stress. So fibrinogens help the blood to clot and PAI-1 helps to stop that clot from dissolving – great when you're under attack but very risky when you're just sitting behind a wheel or at a desk.

So yes, stress can cause heart attacks. Stress leads to high levels of cortisol. High levels of cortisol lead to insulin resistance and insulin resistance can lead to heart disease and, if you do nothing to prevent it, a heart attack. The stress hormones also cause inflammation (see page 47), increasing your chance of heart disease. In fact, one study (*Health for Life* at the Harvard Medical School in 2005) suggested that stress is as likely to cause a heart attack as smoking or high cholesterol.

In a nutshell, fat around the middle is the result of high cortisol and, over time, insulin resistance which means that plaque can build up in the arteries, increasing the risk of heart disease and stroke.

DIABETES

As your cells fail to respond to insulin, your body will always try pumping out more insulin to see if flooding the cells makes any difference. When you're under stress, flooding will make no difference because the message has been sent out to the cells not to respond. This results in a situation where blood sugar levels are high and insulin levels are also high but can't do their job of regulating blood sugar. Over time, this can result in Type 2 or late onset diabetes.

Type 2 diabetes is different from Type 1. Type 1 occurs because of a fundamental problem in the pancreas whereby the cells that are supposed to produce insulin simply can't any more. In this case, blood insulin levels become low (because insulin is not being produced) and blood sugar levels soar dangerously high. In Type 2 diabetes, however, the pancreas produces enough insulin; in fact it produces too much because the cells are not responding to the normal amount.

The major difference between Type 1 and Type 2 diabetes is that in Type 1 the cells in the pancreas that produce insulin are destroyed. This is an anatomical problem. But in Type 2 diabetes, the cells don't work properly. This is a degenerative and preventable problem that has evolved because the body is trying to compensate for a constant state of stress.

A staggering report published by the World Health Organisation (WHO) in October 2005 showed that the accelerating rise in the number of people with Type 2 diabetes could lead to the first reduction in life expectancy for more than 200 years. As Professor Sir George Alberti, the immediate past president of the International Diabetes Federation said, 'This is one of biggest health catastrophes the world has seen.' And, alarmingly, what used to be called 'late onset or middle age' diabetes is now affecting children as young as eleven and twelve.

The WHO report showed that the UK has the fastest growing rate of diabetes in the developed world, with 1.8 million sufferers, a rise of 450 per cent from 1960. A further million are estimated to have diabetes and not even know it.

However, half or more of all diabetes cases could be eliminated if weight gain was prevented and especially weight around the middle of the body.

High Blood Pressure

Research has shown an association between high blood pressure and insulin resistance.[1] High blood pressure (hypertension) happens when the blood exerts too much pressure on the arteries. It is known as the silent killer because it is usually symptom free.

When you are stressed, high cortisol levels prepare you for your fight-or-flight response and your body assumes that it needs a higher blood pressure to cope with this. It holds back sodium (stopping you from excreting it through urine) and this salinates the blood. It is the equivalent of overdosing on salt (sodium chloride) which we know is linked to high blood pressure.

Sodium and potassium, together called electrolytes, normally work in tandem to balance fluid levels in the body. Sodium helps to retain fluid whilst potassium acts as a natural diuretic. When sodium levels are higher, potassium tends to be lower. But potassium – in healthy amounts – is important for lowering blood pressure and also regulating the heart rhythm.

So if your cortisol levels remain high, your blood pressure goes up and you tend to experience water retention, because of the higher sodium. Cortisol also increases the strength of your heart contractions, making the heart work harder as it would under attack.

Cortisol pushes blood around the body diverting it from non-essential areas (such as the digestive system) to places where it thinks it is most needed (such as the arms and legs). It does this by dilating (expanding) blood vessels in some parts of the body and constricting (narrowing) them in other parts. The result is high blood pressure. And as if all this wasn't enough, high cortisol also increases the level of another substance called angiotensin II which is a very strong blood vessel constrictor.

If you have insulin resistance, the excess insulin swimming around in your system will act on the blood vessels making them constrict and get smaller. This makes it is harder for blood to flow and up goes the blood pressure.

Having high blood pressure does not necessarily mean that you have insulin resistance. However, if you do have insulin resistance, there is a good chance that you could develop high blood pressure over time.

As you follow the recommendations in this book, not only will you lose your belly, you will also be controlling or preventing high blood pressure as your levels of cortisol remain normal.

Alzheimer's Disease

Just as high cortisol and then high insulin levels increase the risk of heart disease, a similar process occurs with the blood vessels in the brain. Furring-up combined with continual constriction and dilation causes damage to these blood vessels too, increasing the risk of Alzheimer's and dementia. Research has shown that the risk is higher for women than it is for men, and that the more weight you carry, the higher the risk.[2] If you are obese in middle age, you are 74 per cent more likely to get dementia, as compared with 35 per cent if you are merely overweight.

CANCER

A number of studies have linked high levels of insulin with various cancers, including cancer of the bowel, liver, pancreas, breast, ovary and womb.[3] One study showed that insulin resistance was associated with cancer of the bowel[4] and it has also been shown to increase the risk of breast cancer,[5] womb cancer[6] and ovarian cancer.[7]

We also know that women who are under stress are twice as likely to develop breast cancer as those who are not stressed. A Swedish study of 1,500 women over twenty-four years of age showed that the damaging effects of stress gave them the same risk of breast cancer as those women taking HRT – around 30 per cent. Other factors that could have affected the statistics such as smoking, alcohol intake, age of first pregnancy and age at the menopause were all taken into account.[8]

It has also been suggested that increased body fat is a much stronger predictor of breast cancer risk in women than just measuring their BMI (see page 25). Scientists followed over 12,000 post-menopausal women for eight years and found that those who had gained more than 21kg (3¼ stone) since their menopause had a 75 per cent higher risk of developing breast cancer than women with lower weight gain. Even when all the other risk factors such as smoking, alcohol consumption and HRT use had been taken into account, the body fat percentage was still the most discriminating risk factor.[9]

We also know that where fat is on the body affects the breast cancer risk even more. Doctors at the Harvard School of Public Medicine in America studying 47,000 nurses over a ten-year period found that those who had plump stomachs were 34 per cent more likely to suffer from breast cancer than those who were pear shaped. When the study was narrowed down to just post-menopausal women who had never taken HRT, the apple-shaped women were 88 per cent more likely to get breast cancer.[10]

But how can cancer be linked to problems with cortisol and insulin?

Well, first of all stress affects the immune system, making it less efficient (see page 44) and therefore more susceptible to attack from cancer cells. High cortisol levels reduce the number of 'natural killer' cells that normally help the immune system to identify cancer cells as well as viruses. Cortisol also encourages new blood vessels to form in tumours (angiogenesis) which can stimulate their growth. Cancer cells function in a different way from healthy cells, using glucose as their primary fuel in a process known as anaerobic glycolysis. So if your blood glucose levels are high due to insulin resistance, there will inevitably be excess glucose on which the cancer cells can 'feed'.

This effect of insulin was studied in a trial with over 49,000 post-menopausal women. The researcher found that women with a high carbohydrate and sugar intake had a significantly higher risk of breast cancer. Post-menopausal women who ate foods with a high GI (glycaemic index, see page 59) were 87 per cent more likely to develop breast cancer than those on healthier low-GI diets. The risk was particularly high for women who had used HRT or who did no physical exercise.[11]

Insulin is classed as an anabolic steroid (a 'grower or builder' of cells) and one of the things it does is to encourage cells to mutate. It also stops a process called apoptosis which is literally cell suicide. Healthy cells are normally programmed to die when they have fulfilled their function. If apoptosis is not happening then uncontrolled cell division can take place (just as it does in cancer and in the growth of cancerous tumours).

The other stress link with cancer is the effect of raised cortisol levels on the sex hormones, oestrogen and testosterone. Your adrenal glands produce both male and female sex hormones. In men, the adrenals provide an extra source of testosterone (in addition to that produced by the testes) as well as being their only source of oestrogen. In women, the adrenals provide oestrogen, progesterone and also testosterone.

In women, weight gain around the middle has much to do with a dominance of male hormones. If you have a fractionally higher level of testosterone your body will be more inclined to an apple shape.

OESTROGEN

Oestrogen is not just one hormone, but a group of hormones including oestradiol, oestrone and oestriol.

Oestradiol is produced by the ovaries and is active during our adolescent years. It promotes the deposit of peripheral fat around the hips and thighs – the more 'healthy fat'.

Oestrone is produced by the fat cells from the conversion of male hormones (androgens). This type of oestrogen promotes the storage of fat around the middle.

Oestriol is a weak form of oestrogen. The liver converts oestradiol and oestrone into oestriol to be excreted from the body.

It is interesting to note that Tamoxifen, the drug used to prevent a recurrence of breast cancer, works by blocking oestrogen in the breasts. But the drug used for women who get breast cancer after the menopause is an aromatase inhibitor (called anastrazole) and it stops this conversion of androgens (male hormones) into oestrone.

Oestradiol is usually more dominant before the menopause and causes weight gain in the hips and thighs resulting in a more feminine pear shape. It is not healthy to be overweight but if you're going to put on fat, this is a safer place for it to be.

But thanks to our old friend cortisol, the stress hormones can reduce oestradiol even before the menopause. The stress hormones can affect ovulation (see below) and this in turn reduces the levels of oestradiol being produced by the ovaries. So a number of women will gain weight around the middle of their bodies even before the menopause. Lower levels of oestradiol increase insulin resistance which results in more body fat and this, in turn, promotes more male hormones to be turned into oestrone. And with more oestrone, more fat is stored around the middle. It's a big fat vicious circle.

MORE FAT-AROUND-THE-MIDDLE ISSUES

It is important to be aware of how the killer diseases above can be exacerbated by the damaging effects of cortisol and insulin. You should also be aware, however, of the more subtle changes (below) that could be taking place as a result of your fat distribution.

Irregular periods

If the length of your menstrual cycle is forty days or more, you could have insulin resistance. High levels of insulin could be causing a hormone imbalance which is throwing your cycle out of kilter.[12]

No periods (amenorrhoea)

It is well known that stress can actually cause ovulation and periods to stop in some women.[13] It seems to be Nature's way of protecting a woman from becoming pregnant at a time when she would find it hard to cope. During times of stress, either physical (during crash dieting, for example) or emotional (following bereavement), the body can shut down the reproductive system in order to give the rest of the body the resources it needs to cope.

It is believed that stress interrupts the brain message GnRH (gonadotrophin-releasing hormone) which causes the pituitary gland to release two hormones: FSH (follicle-stimulating hormone) and LH (luteinising hormone). These are both needed to stimulate the ovaries to produce and release eggs. Stress can also increase levels of prolactin, a hormone released by the pituitary gland in high amounts during breastfeeding. It prevents ovulation as a natural means of stopping you from falling pregnant too soon after giving birth.

Premenstrual symptoms

Irritability, aggressive outbursts, palpitations, forgetfulness, anxiety, confusion, inability to concentrate, crying spells, headaches/migraines and food cravings. These are all typical of premenstrual syndrome (PMS). However, they are all also associated with blood sugar fluctuations. In fact, once your blood sugar is under control the symptoms of PMS should be eliminated. Why?

The hormone progesterone normally rises during the second half of the menstrual cycle and progesterone receptors are found all over the body. A receptor acts much like a lock, into which a 'key', in this case, your hormones, must fit. Each lock has a different key; in other words, every receptor uses a different hormone. So progesterone receptors will 'pick up' progesterone for the body to use, in the same way that insulin receptors are supposed to pick up insulin. When blood sugar drops, the body commands adrenaline and cortisol to release sugar stores, but research has found that in the presence of adrenaline the progesterone receptors appear 'blocked'.[14] This means that the body cannot utilise the progesterone, no matter how much of it there may be.

This theory presents a solution to the problem that has been perplexing scientists for decades, namely why women with PMS have the same sex hormone levels as women without. In fact, women with PMS do not have *inadequate* progesterone levels, as was previously thought, it is just that their bodies are not making adequate use of it due to low blood sugar levels and the release of the stress hormones.

As you follow the recommendations in this book, you will start to lose the fat around your middle, and with it your PMS symptoms.

Polycystic ovary syndrome (PCOS)

If you have PCOS your ovaries will be much larger than normal, and will have a tendency to produce a number of undeveloped follicles that appear in clumps, rather like a bunch of grapes. External symptoms include being overweight (especially around the middle), having no or very few periods, being prone to acne, having a problem with unwanted body hair, often on the face, breasts and inside of the legs, and being susceptible to mood swings. If left undiagnosed and untreated PCOS can lead to problems with fertility and recurrent miscarriages.

Blood tests on women with PCOS show higher levels of testosterone, probably due to low levels of a protein called sex hormone-binding globulin (SHBG). Produced by the liver, it binds sex hormones, such as oestrogen and testosterone, and controls how much of them is circulating in the blood at any one time. We know that overweight women have much lower levels of SHBG in their blood resulting in more circulating testosterone and increasingly bad PCOS symptoms, such as excess body hair.[15]

But what does all this have to do with insulin? We know that women with PCOS tend to be insulin resistant and the excess insulin in the body targets the ovaries, urging them to produce more testosterone. It is the surplus of testosterone that causes the 'male' symptoms of excess hair, acne and weight gain around the middle. The insulin also tells the liver to make less SHBG which makes matters worse. High insulin levels mean higher cortisol levels. Cortisol produced when you are under stress also increases insulin levels. This has a knock-on effect on the ovaries stimulating them to produce still more testosterone.

If the true root cause of PCOS (in my opinion, excess cortisol and insulin) is not dealt with successfully then the problem can develop eventually into the full-blown metabolic syndrome, or insulin resistance, involving any or all of the health problems seen on the wheel on page 37. For example, women with PCOS may be seven times more likely to develop diabetes because of problems with blood sugar balance.

If your doctor diagnoses you with PCOS you are most likely to be put on the Pill. New formulations of contraceptive pill contain anti-androgens to control hair growth and acne by preventing excess testosterone from stimulating receptors in the hair and skin. However, the effect does not continue once you stop taking the pills. The Pill helps to produce a regular (albeit artificial) cycle with a withdrawal bleed every month. It regulates your 'periods' for as long as it is taken, but as soon as you stop, the symptoms will recur. You'll be back exactly where you started because nothing will have been done to address the underlying cause. There are also concerns that the Pill could, in fact, be making the problem worse in the longer term, by increasing your insulin resistance.

Although your doctor might offer you a life free from PCOS symptoms with the Pill you should be aware that side effects can include nausea, vomiting, headache, thrombosis, changes in sex drive, depression and breast tenderness. Some doctors might prescribe a drug called Metformin. This has traditionally been used to treat Type 2 or non-insulin-dependent diabetes (NIDDM). But it too comes with possible complications. Side effects can include nausea and an upset stomach. Neither the Pill nor Metformin addresses the underlying cause of the PCOS which really does need to be sorted out not only to get rid of the PCOS and the symptoms but to protect your long-term health.

However, the plan in this book addresses the root cause of PCOS and could provide you with a permanent solution to the distressing symptoms associated with it.

Immune system

During the fight-or-flight response, your immune function will be heightened. This is your body's logical and natural response to any invading bacteria or viruses. But when stress drags on and becomes a constant feature in your day-to-day life the immune function can start to weaken. This is why people in stressful jobs invariably get a cold or the flu as soon as they stop work and go on holiday.

The danger in the long term is that the immune system will break down from overuse, making you susceptible to one infection after another with no resources to fight them off.

What can also happen is that the immune system remains overactive and begins to turn on itself. Your body then starts to attack its own cells as if they were invading organisms. This is known as an auto-immune problem and manifests itself in conditions such as rheumatoid arthritis, lupus erythematosus (an inflammatory condition affecting the skin and internal organs) and Crohn's disease (an inflammatory condition affecting the bowel).

It is now known that the immune systems in women who lead stressful lives are effectively ten years older than they should be. Research has revealed that the immune systems of women who lead stressful lives show an additional ten years of ageing compared with those of unstressed women. This premature ageing of the immune system renders the women more vulnerable to infection and other illnesses.[16]

Ageing

And it's not just the immune system that is 'aged' by stress. We all know people who have been under a lot of stress who end up looking haggard and old before their time.

Cortisol increases oxidative stress which damages neurons, basic cells in the nervous system which transmit electrical impulses and carry information from one part of the body to another. Cortisol also reduces antioxidant enzymes which help to protect cells from damage.

Oxygen which is vital for our survival can also be chemically reactive. It can become unstable, resulting in the 'oxidation' of other molecules, which in turn generates free radicals. Free radicals are chemically unstable atoms that have been linked to health problems including premature ageing, cancer and heart disease. They speed up the ageing process by destroying healthy cells and they can also attack the DNA in the nucleus of a cell, causing cell change (mutation) and cancer.

By reducing your stress response and therefore cortisol you can reduce oxidation in the body and the damage to and premature ageing of our cells.

Insulin and glucose levels in the body may also have an impact on the ageing process. This, the glycation theory of ageing, was introduced in the 1980s and has since been confirmed in a number of studies.[17]

Glycation is the uncontrolled reaction of sugars with proteins, and this happens when glucose and insulin levels are allowed to get out of control. It's a bit like the browning effect on foods when you bake them. If glycation happens, it will create a damaged, 'encrusted' structure in different parts of the body. This process explains why diabetics can be at risk of so many apparently unassociated health problems such as eye disease (cataracts and retinopathy), nerve damage (where sensation is lost in parts of the body) and heart disease. The problems occur if glycation damages the tissues and organs – the protein in cells is damaged, preventing their normal functioning, and membranes and blood vessels are thickened, eventually losing their elasticity. Basically ageing is the accumulation of damaged cells, so the more we can do to reduce the damage to our cells, the slower the ageing process will be and the healthier we will become.

High levels of glucose and high levels of insulin (i.e. insulin resistance) both speed up the damage to cells and that is why it is so important to keep these two substances under control by following the recommendations in this book.

Diabetics tend to age faster than non-diabetics because of cell damage, but keeping tight control over their blood sugar levels can help them to limit the damage.

The same applies if your raised cortisol levels are making you insulin resistant. If you don't do something to bring things back into balance glycation can start to take place even in non-diabetics. This explains why stressed people often look older and have prematurely aged organs.

Tiredness

Whenever you eat your body can either burn your food as energy or store it as fat. But if your cortisol levels are high, the message from your adrenal glands will be to store that food as fat for energy in readiness for fight or flight. So instead of using your food for fuel, your body packs it away in fat stores. This, over time, will inevitably leave you exhausted and susceptible to a real medical condition called TATT – Tired All The Time.

One of the most debilitating aspects of this problem is that you feel not only physically but also mentally tired. Stressed-out people typically get a real slump around three or four o'clock in the afternoon and feel that if they don't have a bar of chocolate or a cup of tea or coffee they'll never get through the afternoon. That is the point at which your blood sugar drops too low and your body asks for a quick fix. But you should resist the temptation to reach for that chocolate bar and instead follow the recommendations in Chapter 4.

Mood swings

There is little doubt that high cortisol levels affect your mood and it is known that people who are depressed have raised cortisol levels. Too much of the chemical in your blood can make you feel anxious, tense and irritable, with a tendency to fly off the handle at the slightest thing. Your body thinks that you are under threat so it gears you up to be aggressive and angry. But on a daily basis, when your life is not really in danger, it is quite easy to explode over something as innocuous as the top having been left off the toothpaste. Following the recommendations in this book will help you to shed the fat around your middle and to keep your moods more stable too.

Inflammation

It is interesting to note that cortisol comes in other guises that you've probably heard of such as cortisone and hydrocortisone. Drug versions of cortisol, known as steroids, are used to treat many illnesses such as rheumatoid arthritis, ulcerative colitis and Crohn's disease, where an anti-inflammatory or immune-suppressing drug is needed.

Research has shown that if your weight sits around your middle it can lead to a low-grade inflammatory effect all over the body. This, in turn, further hampers the body's ability to use insulin because the inflammation blocks insulin, adding to insulin resistance. This has been confirmed by looking at people who have insulin resistance, and they have higher levels of a substance called C-reactive protein, a substance found in the blood when there is inflammation in the body.[18] Researchers at the Joslin Diabetes Centre in the USA found that they could induce diabetes in otherwise healthy animals simply by turning on low-grade inflammation.[19]

Because, as I explained earlier, your fat cells function as a gland, they produce hormones and other substances as do other glands in your body. Unfortunately fat cells produce substances called inflammatory cytokines, which have the effect of pumping up the immune system. This urges the adrenal glands to release more cortisol to calm it down. The excess cortisol in your system then causes more fat to be stored, which then releases more inflammatory cytokines. Round and round it goes once more.

Anybody who has had to take steroids for any reason will know that the side effects tend to be increased appetite and fast weight gain – just like the side effects of too much stress-induced cortisol.

Digestive system

When your body thinks it is under stress and adrenaline and cortisol are released, the energy necessary for digestion is diverted elsewhere so that your

• FOOD ON THE GO •

One in four British workers – about five million people – does not take a full lunch hour and many will even skip lunch. Often people worry that by taking time out to eat they will be giving their bosses a negative impression.

But if you eat on the run, grabbing a sandwich at lunchtime whilst still working at your desk, or rushing off to meet someone and eating the sandwich on the way, you will not digest your food properly. You won't absorb adequately the goodness from that food and will end up feeling bloated and uncomfortable. You may also get loose bowel motions or even diarrhoea as stress hormones continue to relax the rectum muscles.

body can concentrate on saving your life. This means that your levels of stomach acid and digestive enzymes will be lower than they should be.

But stress can do even more to upset your digestive system. In your gut there is a delicate balance of bacteria and yeasts. Some five hundred different species of microflora reside in your gut and there are as many as nine times more bacteria than there are cells in your body. Unfortunately, stress interferes with the levels of beneficial bacteria in the gut, causing them to be lower than they should be. This means that other bacteria and yeasts can grow out of control. A good example of this is the yeast candida albicans which is present in the intestinal tract; in normal, healthy circumstances it does not cause any problems, but if it grows out of control it can cause symptoms such as food cravings (especially for sugar and bread), fatigue, a bloated stomach and flatulence, a 'spaced out' feeling or 'brain fog' and becoming tipsy on a very small amount of alcohol.

Although we tend to think of the gut only in terms of digestion it actually has another role. It acts as an efficient barrier to invading organisms – up to 70 per cent of your immune system is in your gut. So it really is important to maintain good levels of beneficial bacteria (see page 98 for information on how to get enough of them).

Thyroid function

Your adrenal and thyroid gland functions are very much connected and what affects one will usually have a knock-on effect on the other.

Situated in your neck, the thyroid gland helps to control your metabolism. It produces a number of hormones, the most important being thyroxine (or T4). Thyroxine, an inactive hormone, becomes activated when converted to triidothyronine (T3).

The thyroid gland is like a thermostat that regulates your body temperature and tells your body to burn calories and use energy. It is the T3 hormone that makes the metabolism work faster and burn fat. In order for T4 to be converted to T3 the body needs selenium. An underactive thyroid (or hypothyroidism) may be caused by one of two things: either your pituitary gland is not producing thyroid-stimulating hormones (TSH) or your thyroid is not working properly.

If you answer 'yes' to four or more of the following questions, your thyroid gland could be underactive. Your doctor can give you a blood test to establish how well your thyroid is functioning.

- Has your weight gone up gradually over months for no apparent reason?
- Do you often feel cold?
- Are you constipated?
- Are you depressed, forgetful or confused?

- Are you losing hair or is it drier than it used to be?
- Are you having menstrual problems?
- Are you having difficulty in getting pregnant?
- Have you noticed a lack of energy?
- Are you getting headaches?

If a blood test does not show that you have an underactive thyroid, your problem may be a mild one, which could go undetected in a blood test.

The other way to test whether you have low thyroid function is to measure your temperature. If your temperature is too low, it may indicate that you have a sluggish metabolism caused by an underactive thyroid. Cortisol is a key factor in setting the temperature of the body, so with high cortisol levels the body temperature in the morning (basal body temperature) will be low.

Take your temperature once a day for three days. If you are menstruating take your temperature on the second, third and fourth days of the cycle. A woman's body temperature rises after ovulation so it would not give a clear picture if done later in the cycle. If you are not menstruating, take your temperature on any three consecutive days.

Put a thermometer by your bed before you go to sleep (a mercury thermometer is fine but there are some good electronic ones on the market). When you wake, lie still in bed and take your temperature before drinking or visiting the bathroom. Put the thermometer in your armpit and leave it until it bleeps, or if you are using a mercury thermometer, leave it for ten minutes.

If your average temperature over the three days falls below 36.4°C (97.6°F), your thyroid may be under-functioning.

But how does stress fit into this?

High cortisol levels from stress reduce levels of the thyroid hormone T3. This is not a good thing as this is the active thyroid hormone that burns fat. If T3 levels are low, your metabolism inevitably slows down. Added to this, high levels of cortisol will urge your body to break down muscle to provide glucose for your brain and the less muscle you have the slower your metabolism will be (see Chapter 6).

A healthy body converts T4 to T3 (the active thyroid hormone). Under stress, when cortisol levels are high, the conversion of T4 to T3 decreases. The same happens if you are on a diet and restricting your food. Your body assumes that you must be starving so it has to have a way of slowing the metabolism down to preserve those precious fat stores. It's infuriating, but it's only your body thinking about your survival.

High cortisol also inhibits the messenger hormone – thyroid stimulating hormone (TSH) – which is sent from the pituitary gland. With less TSH, the thyroid gland produces less thyroxine T4.

Memory and concentration

Higher levels of cortisol are associated with poor memory and concentration as they can damage the memory centre (hippocampus) of the brain by depriving it of the glucose it needs to function efficiently. Even short periods of stress, say two weeks of raised cortisol levels, can cause brain cell connections to shrivel up.[20] This helps to explain why you might, when stressed, spend hours looking for your car keys, or walk into a room and then wonder what on earth you went in there for! The good news is, however, that these effects are reversible, and the connections can grow back if cortisol levels are reduced.

Skin changes

Insulin makes the skin grow in different ways. This can be in the form of skin tags (tiny pieces of excess skin, like floppy moles, hanging off your body), for example. These can be a sign that you are struggling with blood sugar swings and that you could be insulin resistant because excess insulin has stimulated the skin to grow. Excess insulin can also change the appearance of the skin so that it looks a little like black velvet. The process, called acanthosis nigricans, makes the skin look dirty in patches but the shadowing will not wash off. You should consult your doctor if you have this discolouration because, very rarely, it can be cancerous. But if you are given the all-clear your skin will return to normal if you sort out your insulin resistance and follow the recommendations in this book.

As you can see from all the health changes discussed in this chapter, it is important to get rid of that fat around the middle, not only because you are going to look better, but also because it is going to have a significant positive impact on your health, now and in the future.

• Chapter 4 •

What and How to Eat

Simple dietary tricks to teach your body to burn fat rather than store it

There is absolutely no doubt that a good diet is extremely important in terms of both your health and your weight. However, unless you address the spiralling stress cascade that creates and holds on to the fat around your middle, even the best diet in the world will not help you. As we have seen in earlier chapters your body has been holding on to that fat around your middle because it thinks it is under attack, so to correct that pattern you will have to change the fundamental message that your body is receiving.

Altering your eating patterns in order to shift the weight is an important start. Your eating habits may be telling your body that it is under stress. If you restrict your diet or cut calories your body inevitably thinks there is a famine out there and that causes stress. It will slow down your metabolism to hold on to your precious fat stores and if your blood sugar levels fluctuate your body will also be releasing adrenaline (see below), the same hormone it releases when you are under stress. This also encourages your body to store fat.

The solution is to find a way of eating that tells your body that all is well, reassuring it that there is no 'threat'. You need to change your body's underlying biochemistry, not embark on a weight-loss diet.

Blood Sugar Swings

You are currently stuck in a vicious circle of stress hormones and blood sugar swings. The two important points to remember are:

- Adrenaline and cortisol are released when you are under stress.
- Adrenaline and cortisol are released when your blood sugar drops.

Your body is trying in both cases to release your sugar stores. It does this when you are stressed to give you instant energy to fight or run. And it does this when your blood sugar drops because it needs to correct the low level. Although your body does not care why the adrenaline and cortisol are being released, the damaging effect on your health is the same.

Think of your blood sugar fluctuations as a rollercoaster.

The rollercoaster track is your blood sugar: insulin is produced as it rises and as it falls adrenaline and cortisol are released.

Blood sugar rollercoaster

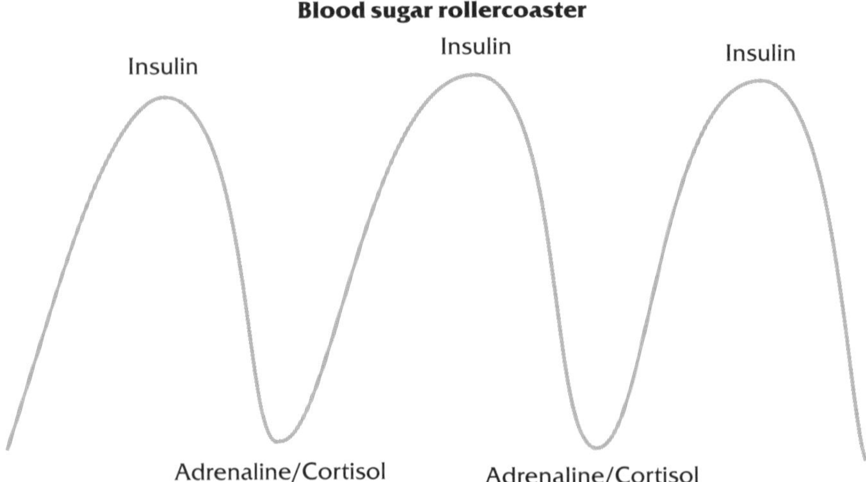

As you eat or drink your blood sugar goes up and insulin is released. If you are eating refined foods like sugar, white bread, cakes and biscuits or stimulant drinks like coffee, tea or cola, they will hit your bloodstream quickly. More insulin will be released to deal with this sudden rise in blood sugar. Once dealt with, the blood sugar levels will drop, but because you've triggered the release of so much insulin, the levels will drop too low and you'll soon feel hungry again. The higher the blood sugar highs, the lower the lows will be afterwards.

At the drop your body will register a low blood sugar level – hypoglycaemia – and do two things. It will give you a physical craving for a cup of coffee or a bar of chocolate – a quick fix to bring the blood sugar up again. It will also trigger the adrenal glands to produce more adrenaline and cortisol to help it to release stores of sugar to correct the low level.

Hypoglycaemia can leave you with: irritability, aggressive outbursts, palpitations, lack of sex drive, crying spells, dizziness, anxiety, confusion, forgetfulness, inability to concentrate, fatigue, insomnia, headaches and muscle cramps.

I have seen women in my clinic who were diagnosed with panic attacks because they were experiencing these symptoms. A severe episode of hypoglycaemia can look like a panic attack because the body literally thinks it is under attack and so it releases stress hormones. One woman I treated would go into a supermarket but have to leave her trolley full of food and run out of the store as her hypoglycaemia hit. She would be literally running for her life, her body in flight-or-fight mode, forcing her to do something. By getting her blood sugar under control, her 'panic attacks' disappeared.

The best way to get the message to your body that it is not under stress so that it produces less adrenaline and also less cortisol (ultimately responsible for the fat around your middle), you need to control your blood sugar levels.

COMFORT OR STRESS EATING

We are all different. Some women lose their appetite and lose weight under stress, whilst others eat more. Research has found that women who produce more cortisol (even when not under stress) tend to be 'comfort eaters'. One study took fifty-nine pre-menopausal women and gave them both a stress session and a non-stress session on different days. The women who produced more cortisol in the stress session ate more calories compared with those who produced normal levels of cortisol. They also found themselves drawn to sweeter foods. In the non-stress session, all the women (high and low cortisol producers) ate similar amounts of food. Stress, it seems, induced the women who produced more cortisol not only to eat more but to go for the more sugary foods.[1]

Although we now understand that the body does this in order to refuel after a stress event it is not an inevitable process. You can break out of the vicious circle and regain your waist once more. It's really very simple, and here is how.

MY OH-SO-SIMPLE NINE-STEP EATING PLAN

1. Stop dieting (yes, really!) and don't count calories.
2. Eat little and often.
3. Don't skip breakfast.
4. Eliminate all sugar and refined carbohydrates from your life.
5. Add protein to each meal.
6. Eat essential fats.
7. Don't eat on the run.
8. Watch what you drink.
9. Change the way in which you think about food.

1. Stop dieting

No one enjoys dieting. It's difficult, frustrating, often expensive and anti-social. So now here's the definitive excuse for never having to diet again. Diets do not work. It's a fact, and it's as true now as it was in 1999 when I wrote the book *Natural Alternatives to Dieting*. Up to a third of all women who diet end up weighing as much as a stone after they diet than they did before. The diet industry is big business and, unbeknown to you, it actually wants you to fail. You can buy meal replacement drinks, slimming pills, low-fat food, low-carb snack bars and low-calorie products but if they all worked as well as they claimed, you would only need them for a short while and the manufacturers would go out of business.

Dieting – defined as energy in = less than energy out, in other words a severe restriction of food – is a biologically unnatural state. It simply does not give your body enough fuel to do the jobs it needs to do. Your mind and body hear alarm bells and go into survival mode: holding on to the weight you have, slowing your metabolism and telling you to eat, eat, eat.

Here is a classic example. You have been on a crash diet for a couple of days and everything seems to be going well. Then your friend comes round with a cake. Being sociable, you decide that a little bit won't hurt. But once you start eating, it is as if you can't stop. For your body the diet was like a trip through the desert and now that it has stumbled across an oasis it stocks up with as much as possible. Your compulsion to eat almost the entire cake is not a sign that you are weak willed or piggish, it is simply an irrepressible biological urge over which you have very little control. Your body thought you were starving, and to some extent you were. So if you really want to lose weight, and specifically tummy fat, then restricting your food intake is the last thing you should do.

Yo-yo dieting

Many women tend to yo-yo diet – they go on a diet for a couple of weeks, lose some weight, then go back to eating normally. The weight goes back on and they find that they are heavier than they were before starting the diet. So they embark on an even stricter diet, then stop and even more weight piles on.

Yo-yo dieting is very common but there are two problems associated with this pattern. Firstly, it disrupts your metabolism. Each time you restrict your food intake your metabolism drops, then when you return to your normal diet, you will be eating it on a slower metabolism as your body takes time to readjust. As a result, when you come off a diet, you'll gain more weight than before. This simple change in the body's biochemistry can happen on a daily basis. I see women in the clinic who don't eat lunch and just have a cup of coffee. They assume that if they are missing out the calories at lunch they must lose weight. But they don't. And they would have to be superhuman to be able to resist overeating in the evening when their body is crying out for food.

Over the course of a day, the body registers that food is in short supply so slows down the metabolism. Your body does not know whether you are going to eat in six hours or six days, so it errs on the side of caution. When you sit down to eat your long-awaited evening meal the stress response caused by the perceived starvation means the body does its utmost to store as much of that meal as fat as it possibly can. Peppering your day with appetite-suppressing cups of coffee or cans of cola only makes matters worse because the caffeine releases adrenaline and cortisol, so encouraging your body to store even more fat.

When you return to eating normally again after a diet the weight lost (a combination of water, muscle and, if you're lucky, a bit of fat) will go back on as fat only. The body has been starved and is programmed to try to store up fat quickly in case another 'famine' is just around the corner. That explains why it is so common to gain even more weight (fat) after a diet. And so the cycle goes on.

You must lose fat, not just weight

This is where the second problem with yo-yo dieting comes in. However satisfying it is to stand on the scales at the end of a week and see that the pounds have fallen away, it is not realistic. If you lose weight quickly, a quarter of that weight loss will be made up of water, muscle and bone – not the fat you so want to lose. Fast weight loss might be exciting, but you cannot physically lose more than 450–900g (1–2lb) of fat a week, so give yourself a break.

On a crash diet your starving body will use muscle tissue as fuel. This is never a good idea, not least because muscle actually helps you to burn fat, so the more muscle you have the better. Also, your body converts muscle into glucose for energy when you crash diet, and this also has the advantage of decreasing energy expenditure because muscle is metabolically active and in itself uses up energy. But your body can use any muscle including your heart.

That's why it is so important to keep up a good level of activity when you want to burn fat, because muscles are metabolically active and help you to burn off fat much more quickly.

If your crash diet seems to be working and you manage to lose as much as 10 per cent of your body weight, your metabolism adapts by slowing down its rate of energy expenditure by as much as 15 per cent. This is how humans manage to survive for months without food. It also helps to explain why on a low-calorie diet it is often so difficult to shed those last four or five kilograms. In spite of your best efforts, your body is slowing everything down to match the food intake in a desperate bid to hold on to those last few kilograms. That is why it is so important to lose weight (fat) very slowly and to keep the metabolism at a healthy (high) level throughout.

What is a calorie?

A calorie is a unit of heat and is the energy-producing property of food. It was traditionally thought that if the number of the calories going into the body were less than the calories being used by physical activity, you would lose weight. But we now know that this does not seem to work for everybody. You probably know people who are active, do not eat very much but still can't lose weight.

All calories are not equal and their effect on your weight gain or loss will depend on whether they come from fats, proteins or carbohydrates.

Furthermore, energy is needed to digest food. This is the thermic effect of food which means that some of the calories in food are used to digest it. Some foods, for example lettuce, are classed as having negative calories because more calories are needed to digest them than the amount of calories they provide. The thermic effect of food lasts for about three hours after you eat.

Protein, carbohydrates and fats have different thermic effects. Eating protein burns off far more energy (it takes about 20 per cent of your body's energy to metabolise), than eating carbohydrate (10 per cent) and fat (2 per cent). So what you eat is just as important as how much.

Whilst you will not lose weight if you overeat and don't burn it off, I am very much against counting calories and urge you to stop thinking about food as a set of numbers (whether calories or GI). Instead, look at portion size and, certainly when it comes to your two bigger meals of the day (lunch and dinner), try to reduce the amount on your plate by about a quarter. It is very important to become more aware of what you are eating and, specifically, how much of it.

2. Eat little and often

This is an extremely important life change. The idea is to convince your body that food is abundant, that it does not need to store extra fat and that it can burn off any excess that is already stored. If you go for longer than three hours without food your body will start to make preparations for going into survival mode. Stress levels rise, out comes the cortisol, and, with it, the instructions to hold on to fat and break down muscle to provide fuel.

You may start to feel light-headed or irritable as your blood sugar drops and that is the point at which you will typically reach out for a quick boost in the form of a cup of coffee and a biscuit. At the same time, your adrenal glands will release both adrenaline and cortisol to urge the liver to produce more glucose.

It's easy to become a healthy grazer instead. If you train yourself to eat something small every three hours you will be sending your body the message that it is not under stress, that it can kick your metabolism up a notch and, if it likes, plunder the old fat stores for energy too! A study in the *New England Journal of Medicine*[2] showed that simply by switching to a regime of eating every three hours you can reduce your body's damaging cortisol levels by 17 per cent in just two weeks. Participants in the study ate exactly the same amount of food as normal but instead of eating it in three big meals, they divided it into smaller, more frequent meals. This also ties in with the mechanism of the thermic effect of food (see above) which lasts for about three hours after eating, so as you eat again your body will be burning off more fat as it switches to digestion mode again.

When you switch to eating little and often you'll notice three big differences:

- You will get your energy back. Because your blood sugar is stable (you are effectively topping it up every three hours) your energy levels will also be stable and there will be no more rollercoaster highs and lows.
- Your cravings for sweet foods and refined carbohydrates will stop. Again, because your blood sugar does not drop, your body will no longer have to ask you for a quick fix. It is as easy as that. Whereas previously you would have had to have been superhuman to resist the physiological urge to correct your blood sugar dips, once your blood sugar is steady, you'll be amazed at how easy it will be to resist that piece of chocolate cake.
- As the blood sugar steadies, so will the mood swings. Because you've come off that rollercoaster of irritability, aggressive outbursts, crying spells, anxiety and tension your body will no longer think it is under attack. As your cortisol levels reduce you will automatically start to feel happier and calmer inside. The human body is a marvellous and complex device and you cannot separate body from mind. As you change what is going on physically, your emotions and feelings will also change.

Eating little and often is simple. Just make sure you eat three meals a day – breakfast, lunch and dinner – plus a snack mid-morning and one mid-afternoon, leaving no longer than three hours between each meal or snack. (See pages 141–155 for meal and snack suggestions.)

3. Don't skip breakfast

Many experts – myself included! – believe that breakfast is the most important meal of the day.

Many people are so stressed in the morning, rushing to get kids off to school and themselves ready for work, that they will just grab a cup of coffee (often with sugar) and go on their way. However, in doing so they are setting themselves up for failure. Remember the rollercoaster: up goes the blood sugar, out pumps the excess insulin, giving the message, loud and clear, to store that fat around the middle.

If you miss breakfast completely your body starts to attack the muscles, breaking them down for fuel. Muscles are metabolically active and help to burn fat so you really don't want this to happen. With no breakfast inside you, blood sugar will drop within a couple of hours, adrenaline and cortisol will kick in to try to correct the balance and you'll be looking for a quick fix.

I can't stress enough the importance of making time for breakfast. Try to allow yourself just ten to fifteen minutes to sit down and eat a bowl of porridge or cereal (sugar free), or a piece of rye toast with pure fruit jam. Train yourself to do this – it is so essential.

You may not be a big fan of porridge but it can give you a steady rise in blood sugar (not the instant varieties) and to pep it up you could add some spices. Cinnamon is especially helpful as it improves the transport of glucose into the cells and has been known to lower glucose levels in Type 2 diabetes. Cinnamon is also thermogenic which means that it helps to burn off fat.[3] Turmeric is an interesting spice too in that it helps to control inflammation and we know that inflammation is connected to fat around the middle, so adding this spice to other meals could be beneficial.

4. Eliminate all sugar and refined carbohydrates from your life

The aim of the game, as we know, is to control your natural stress response so that your body gets the message to stop storing fat around the middle of your body. You can effectively cut out all dietary stress by simply swapping your usual diet for eating little and often. But you can take another big step in the right direction by avoiding any foods that make your blood sugar rise quickly.

To do this properly, you need to eliminate from your diet any foods that are digested very quickly. You could do this by religiously adhering to one of the increasingly popular GI diets, but, in my opinion, they are far too complicated. There is a much easier way.

The simple way to eat the 'right' foods

In a nutshell, the faster a food is digested, the sooner it hits your bloodstream and the bigger the stress response is as a result.

Think of the difference between putting paper on a fire or coals. The paper will burn quickly with a big show of flames, but it does not give out much heat and burns so quickly that before long you have to put more paper on the fire. Coal, on the other hand, takes longer to heat up but gives you a steady level of heat over a much longer period.

In dietary terms, your aim is to eat food that acts in the same way as coal, not paper, no matter how attractive that option can sometimes be! Refined and processed foods are as paper to the body's fire; natural whole foods are coal.

The more a food is refined (i.e. the more natural substances are removed) the faster the hit on your bloodstream will be. If you eat more food in its natural form, your blood sugar will be much more steady.

A good example is the difference between white and wholemeal bread. Because white bread has been stripped of fibre it rushes through the digestive system causing insulin levels to rise. Wholemeal bread, on the other hand, is made from the whole grain ground down and includes the outer husk. Because of the fibre in wholemeal bread the body takes a while to absorb its goodness, slowing its progress through your system, and giving your body a chance to react in a natural, stress-free way.

GI: CONFUSED? YOU SOON WILL BE!

The glycaemic index (GI) was conceived by Dr David Jenkins in 1981 in a paper he wrote for the *American Journal of Clinical Nutrition* suggesting that not all carbohydrates were broken down at the same rate and that those that were broken down more quickly would cause a high rise in blood sugar. Jenkins initially advocated the use of the GI for the management of Type 1 diabetes and later for problems with high cholesterol and triglycerides.[4]

Glucose was given a GI of 100 because it causes the quickest rise in blood sugar, and 50g (2oz) of various carbohydrates were then compared with 50g (2oz) of glucose. According to some of the initial results ice cream registered as a better food for diabetics than wholewheat bread! However, in 1983, other researchers compared the same carbohydrates and got different results. Some experts believe that the results depend on the person's level of blood sugar at the time of the test. Another flaw is that carbohydrates were being tested in isolation, unlike 'real-life' eating.

By 1988 the standard against which all foods were compared had been changed from sugar to white bread, but, in time, doubts began to surface again about the accuracy of the GI. The problem is that a number of factors can affect the reproducibility of a GI measure, including the ripeness of the food; the physical form of the food (mashing a 2.5cm (1in) cube of potato increases its GI by 25 per cent); variability within food classes (e.g. different shapes of pasta, consistency, cooking etc.). So the GI is not very helpful. It tells us how quickly that carbohydrate turns into sugar, but does not say how much carbohydrate a particular quantity of food contains. This explains such bizarre contradictions as chocolate (GI 48) having a lower GI than watermelon (GI 72).

Enter GL

A new measure called the Glycaemic Load (GL) was introduced to overcome some of the problems with GI. GL takes into account how much of the carbohydrate is in the food. The real impact on your blood glucose levels will be determined by both the quality (GI) and the quantity (GL) of the carbohydrate.

People were even avoiding carrots on the GI diet because they had a GI of 48, the same as chocolate. But the GL of carrots is 3.9 compared to 14 for chocolate.

So, it's best to forget GI and think GL. Or is it? Scientists have moved the theory on and are now suggesting another measure, which they call Glycaemic Glucose Equivalent (GGE). This supposedly has more 'meaning' than GL.[5]

It all gets very confusing and I am in no doubt that before long another concept will emerge to supersede the GGE.

So my recommendation to you is to forget the lot! Counting calories, fat grams, GI, GL and now GGE can drive you insane. There is a much simpler way to eat without carrying around charts and looking up data on every mouthful.

Slice for slice, wholemeal bread contains four times as much fibre, more than three times as much zinc and almost twice as much iron as white bread. The carbohydrates in wholemeal bread are broken down slowly over several hours, like the coals in the fire, and so do not give any sudden flooding of sugars into the bloodstream. Also this gradual release helps you to feel full for longer, suppressing your appetite and stopping you craving sweet foods because you are not on the blood sugar rollercoaster.

A study of 459 healthy people at Tufts University in Boston in 2004 showed that those who consumed the most white bread had the biggest increases in waist measurement. The girth of white bread eaters increased by nearly a centimetre (half an inch) a year (the study was conducted over three years) – three times more than those who habitually ate wholemeal bread.

Recent research has shown that eating slow-release foods (such as wholemeal bread) not only helps to balance your blood sugar but also benefits your heart and reduces or prevents diabetes. This makes complete sense knowing what we now do about insulin resistance (see page 30).[6]

Interestingly, whole grains also contain 'enzyme inhibitors' – substances which delay the digestion of starch and sugar, stop the increase in blood glucose levels and so effectively reduce the glycaemic response. They have a similar action to the drugs given to help control Type 2 diabetes (alpha glucosidase inhibiting medications), slowing the release of glucose into the blood through the delayed digestion of carbohydrates.

Carbohydrates – and everything you really need to know about them

Most foods contain a mixture of carbohydrates, fats and proteins, all in different combinations.

BEWARE OF BRAN

Don't think you can eat white bread instead of wholemeal and simply compensate by adding bran to other meals.

Bran is technically a refined food because it is stripped away from the whole grain and sold on its own. Bran contains substances called 'phytates' which, once consumed, bind valuable minerals, attracting calcium, zinc, magnesium amongst others like a magnet. These minerals, essential for your general health, are then excreted with the bran from the digestive tract. Ironically, although bran is often used to overcome constipation, it can irritate the digestive system causing bloating and irritable bowel-like symptoms.

It is far better to eat bran in the form that Nature intended, as part of the whole grain – as in wholemeal bread.

FIBRE

People often tend to think of fibre only in relation to the bowels and alleviating constipation. But it also plays an important part in helping to remove that fat around the middle. The fibre in whole foods helps to control your blood sugar swings (and so reduce the amount of cortisol being released) by slowing the rate of food leaving the stomach. Slower digestion means that you do not get a fast release of sugar into the bloodstream and no high levels of insulin are pumped out. Fibre can also give you a sense of fullness which helps with appetite control by making you feel less hungry.

There are two main types of fibre:

- soluble – found in fruits, oats, vegetables and beans
- insoluble – found in whole grains and nuts

Soluble fibre is better for managing blood sugar swings as it has the biggest impact on controlling insulin.[7] Soluble fibre also helps to regulate cholesterol because it binds with some of the cholesterol and fat in the food you eat and excretes it out of the body.

Insoluble fibre is known as roughage and helps to move food through your intestines.

Carbohydrates are starches and sugars and the easiest way to think about them is to split them into two groups – fast releasing and slow releasing.

Fast-releasing carbohydrates will cause a rapid rise in blood sugar, followed by a drop and the subsequent release of stress hormones. So any food that has sugar added to it becomes fast releasing. Look out for sugar on food labels and take note of its many guises including:

- fructose – fruit sugar
- glucose – body blood sugar, fast acting
- dextrose – sugar from cornstarch, chemically identical to glucose
- lactose – milk sugar
- maltose – made from starch
- sucrose – common table sugar, made from sugar cane or beet

Whatever the name, these are all sugar and, as such, will contribute to insulin resistance and weight gain around your middle. Food companies are obliged to list ingredients in order of quantity – so if all sugars were grouped under the word 'sugar' this word would appear first on very many labels. However, they cleverly split the sugar into its different forms (sucrose, dextrose etc.) to spread the perceived sugar load and shift it a little further down the list.

Be vigilant. Sugar is added to savoury foods like tinned vegetables, baked beans, tomato ketchup, soups and even pasta sauces where you might least expect it. A small pot of fruit yogurt, even a 'healthy' organic live fruit yogurt can contain as much as eight teaspoons of sugar.

If you really want to get rid of that weight around the middle you need to cut out all sugars completely, except for the odd bit on special occasions.

As I said before, any food that has been refined will be fast releasing (white bread, white rice, biscuits and cakes). And some fast-releasing foods like biscuits and cakes have a double effect because they combine sugar and white flour.

Fruit is a healthy food and gives us many valuable vitamins and minerals, especially antioxidants which help to protect cells from damage and slow the ageing process. But fruit is also high in fructose. So in order to get your blood sugar under control it is better to limit your fruit intake to the slow-releasing types in the table below.

Bananas and grapes are among the fastest releasing, so don't eat a lot of them and always have a protein with them like nuts or seeds. When a fruit is dried sugar levels are more concentrated so eat raisins sparingly or combine them with a protein for a snack (as nuts and raisins perhaps). I would recommend avoiding fruit juice for the first four weeks and then only enjoying it in diluted form and with food. There may well be as many as eight oranges in a glass of orange juice but you'd be far better off eating the oranges themselves so the fibre helps slow the rate of digestion.

It is better to avoid starchy potatoes and sweet potatoes for the first three months until you've got your fat distribution under control.

Slow-releasing carbohydrates	**Fast-releasing carbohydrates**
Grains (whole wheat, rye, oats including porridge, brown rice, barley, maize, quinoa, millet)	Refined grains (white flour, cakes, biscuits, white bread, pastries, instant porridge, white rice)
Beans (lentils, kidney beans, soya, etc.)	White and brown sugar, glucose, honey, maple syrup
Vegetables (plus buckwheat which is not a grain but part of the rhubarb family)	Potatoes and sweet potatoes
Fruits, especially any berries, cherries, apples, pears and citrus	Bananas, dried fruit, grapes and fruit juice

Wheat

Wheat is high in amylopectin – the most common form of starch. This is faster releasing and does not have the same positive effect on insulin as amylose (see page 63). So although wholemeal bread is better for you than white bread, if you

Resistant Starch

Not all whole grains behave in the same way in the body. Resistant starch – so called because it is resistant to stomach acid and digestive enzymes – reaches the large intestine essentially intact. So it manages to escape digestion and absorption in the small intestine. It almost behaves like fibre, providing bulk for the bowel motion and fuel for the beneficial bacteria.

Amylose – found in legumes (beans) and oats – is a resistant starch and has a significant positive impact on slowing down the insulin response.[8]

want to remove the weight more quickly it is better to avoid wheat most of the time and go for breads and pasta made with other grains such as rye and corn.

Wheat also contains a protein called gluten which forms a sticky substance in the digestive system (very much like flour and water glue). Because gluten is sticky and difficult to digest it encourages the growth of unfriendly bacteria which can produce toxic substances and gas. The extreme form of this problem is coeliac disease, an intolerance to the gluten found in grains such as wheat, rye, barley and oats. Coeliac disease sufferers are found to have white blood cells in their gut lining which are programmed to 'see' gluten as a foreign substance and so reject it. Coeliac disease is characterised by weight loss and diarrhoea and many essential vitamins and minerals do not get absorbed. It is important to see your doctor for a diagnosis if you suspect that this might be the problem.

Modern wheat has been grown to be high in gluten to make mass production easier and cheaper. If you get a lot of digestive problems like indigestion, flatulence, bloating, constipation or diarrhoea then it is worth eliminating wheat for a week to see if it makes any difference. Watch out for wheat added to soups, sauces or gravies (it may appear as 'starch' on the label and will most certainly be refined). If you find that you feel more comfortable without wheat you could try a grain called spelt (which is far lower in gluten). Known as 'the grandparent' of modern wheat, spelt is digested perfectly well by many people who can't tolerate wheat.

Carbohydrates and your health

So what does all this mean in terms of your health? We know that women with a high carbohydrate consumption carry a higher risk of breast cancer. Women who obtained 57 per cent or more of their total calories from carbohydrates were more than twice as likely to get breast cancer.[9] The sugars sucrose and fructose showed the strongest association with breast cancer risk. The higher level of insulin triggered by the sugar promotes cell division and also leads to higher levels of oestrogen in the body. In this study fibre was linked to a lower risk as it slowed the absorption of carbohydrates.

• THE TRUTH ABOUT FRUCTOSE •

Fructose in powdered form comes not from fruit but is a highly refined product from corn. Fructose was always thought to be safe for diabetics because it does not cause the rapid rise in blood sugar that sucrose does. Unfortunately, however, it has other negative effects. The body treats fructose differently from sucrose and shunts it directly to the liver for the formation of fats. Thus, it boosts blood levels of cholesterol and triglycerides and also stimulates the production of insulin and cortisol. Although it does not cause a rise in blood sugar it can still cause insulin resistance.

This is very different from eating the fructose in fruit where it comes with fibre and all the other naturally occurring vitamins and minerals in that food.

We could talk about slow- and fast-releasing carbohydrates as being 'good' and 'bad' carbohydrates but I would like to suggest that we think of them as healthy and unhealthy carbohydrates which is basically what they are. The unhealthy carbohydrates will make you fat around the middle together with all the associated health risks (see Chapter 3). Healthy carbs will not. This has been clearly shown in animals where two groups of rats were fed on nearly identical diets, containing 69 per cent carbohydrates. One group was given slow-releasing carbohydrates whilst the other group had fast-releasing carbohydrates. After eighteen weeks, the fast-releasing carb rats had 71 per cent more body fat, much of it concentrated around the middle of their bodies. They created apple-shaped rats! A second study in mice showed even more marked results, with the fast-releasing carb group having 93 per cent more body fat than the slow-releasing group.[10]

The bottom line is that your body does need carbohydrates – it is, after all, the most preferred source of fuel – but it is the quality of the carbohydrates you eat and their balance with protein in any meal that is so important.

Your brain runs on carbohydrates and that is why you can feel depressed, moody and unable to think straight (brain fog) if you are not eating enough of them. So I would never recommend a low-carbohydrate diet. It is just that in Western society we have become used to eating a lot of carbohydrates and unfortunately the wrong type.

Restricting your carbohydrates too much over a few weeks has been shown to affect thyroid function by lowering the hormones, so affecting your metabolism. Too few carbohydrates will also cause your blood sugar to drop and your body to release adrenaline to raise your blood glucose. This will result in high cortisol levels. As we have discussed previously, high cortisol will tell your body to store weight around your middle and will also have a further impact on your thyroid function. You will then be stuck in a vicious circle.

ARTIFICIAL SWEETENERS – AS BAD AS SUGAR

'Low-sugar', 'diet' or 'low-calorie' foods and drinks usually contain chemical sweeteners, such as aspartame. These sweeteners also appear in crisps, ice lollies, sauces, instant noodles and some medicines (check labels carefully).

It is a common misconception, however, that artificial sweeteners help you to lose and control your weight. Studies have shown that people who regularly use artificial sweeteners tend to gain weight through increased appetite.[11]

Many kinds of artificial sweeteners are available, including saccharin (the oldest), cyclamate, acesulfame-K, sucralose and aspartame. Aspartame is one of the most widely used artificial sweeteners.

Aspartame is 180 times sweeter than sugar and can lead to binge eating and cravings. It has also been linked to mood swings and depression because it alters the levels of the brain chemical serotonin.[12] Depression is often treated with SSRI drugs (selective serotonin reuptake inhibitors). These are designed to optimise the use of serotonin, helping to lift mood and reduce appetite, whilst aspartame works in exactly the opposite way.

However, aspartame is also worrying for other reasons and, in America the Aspartame Toxicity Information Centre (www.holisticmed.com/aspartame) has been set up, because of concerns that aspartame may be causing more serious health problems. When digested it releases methanol and two amino acids, aspartic acid and phenylalanine, into the body. Methanol converts to formaldehyde – a toxin classed in the same group of drugs as cyanide and arsenic! – and then to formate or formic acid.[13] Amino acids are fundamental constituents of all proteins, and they interact with each other. Amino acids are normally ingested in small quantities in proteins, and in combination with other amino aids. In the case of aspartame, however, aspartic acid and phenylalanine are being ingested on their own, and in much larger quantities. The result is that they can unbalance the metabolism of amino acid in the brain.[14] In other words, they affect the way our brains use amino acids.

Fresh fears were raised about aspartame in 2005 as the European Food Safety Authority was reviewing the results of a large study from Italy showing that aspartame could cause lymphomas and leukaemia in female laboratory animals in doses similar to the usual daily intake for humans.

There are also concerns that aspartame might be addictive, and that people who drink a large number (three to four cans) of diet soft drinks every day, or regularly chew sugar-free gum, may experience withdrawal symptoms if they try to stop. The following symptoms are all associated with regular aspartame consumption: mood swings, memory loss, numbness and tingling in the arms and legs, headaches, depression, skin problems, such as urticaria (a bit like hives) and rashes, seizures and convulsions, eye problems, nausea and vomiting.

I always advise patients to avoid any foods or drinks containing artificial sweeteners but to do this effectively you will need to read the very small print on all labels as sweeteners can crop up in savoury as well as sweet foods, whether they are branded 'diet' or otherwise.

5. Add protein to each meal

Protein is a vital part of the diet because it is the basic building block for all the cells, muscles and bones as well as the hair, skin and nails. Proteins are made from twenty-five amino acids, eight of which are called 'essential' because they must be obtained from food, unlike the other seventeen which are made naturally by the body. Because your muscles are made of protein you need to ensure that you are getting enough protein to maintain your muscle mass – don't forget that muscles help to shift the weight around the middle because they increase your metabolism which, in turn, burns fat.

Protein should be included in each meal as it slows down the rate at which the stomach empties its food into the next part of the digestive tract, so slowing the passage of the carbohydrates with it. As soon as you add a protein (be it animal or vegetable) to a carbohydrate you change it into a slow-releasing carbohydrate, which is a very good thing. Adding protein can be as simple as sprinkling nuts and seeds on your porridge for breakfast in the morning. (See the meal suggestions in Chapter 10 for ideas.)

As with most things balance is important and that includes the balance between proteins, carbohydrates and fats. And, of course, eating protein with every meal goes right against the principles of food combining (or food *un*combining as I like to call it).

Food combining is based on the belief that protein and carbohydrates should be eaten at separate meals because the two need different enzymes to be digested effectively. It is said that if they are eaten together the resultant undigested food is stored firstly in the intestines, leading to fermentation causing bloating and flatulence, then, if it is not properly digested and used as energy, it is stored as fat.

Although there seems to be no scientific basis for this regime people do lose weight on it. This could be because they reduce portion size unconsciously. I am very clear, however, that food combining is not good for anyone with an apple shape because it will only make the blood sugar fluctuations worse – especially after the carbohydrate-only meals.

Protein helps in the control of insulin because it slows the rate of digestion. It also encourages the production of glucagon, the fat-burning hormone. Glucagon, like insulin, is produced by the pancreas, but it works in the opposite way to insulin and increases blood glucose by encouraging the body to burn fat for energy.

But however important protein may be, a high-protein or protein-only diet is not, in my opinion, to be recommended. In the long term, this type of diet is not only unhealthy, but can also be dangerous. Again, it is a question of balance.

The problem is, when the body is starved of carbohydrates it looks for energy in its glycogen stores. Because 4g of water cling to every gram of glycogen, you can appear to lose a lot of weight very quickly on a low-carb diet. But the immediate weight loss will always be water, not fat. Only when the glycogen stores are completely depleted will the body start to dissolve fat cells.

If you eat nothing but protein your body can go into an abnormal metabolic state called 'ketosis'. Because there is not enough carbohydrate the body has to use fat for fuel. Ketones are produced during starvation and in diabetes mellitus and when this happens the body is literally eating itself in order to stay alive. Not only is fat used for energy but muscle is also broken down. Ketones produce side effects too, including bad breath, poor concentration, mood swings and bad memory. I have also seen a number of women in my clinic who used a ketogenic diet to lose weight and lost a massive amount of hair after stopping the diet.

You may feel that these are small prices to pay for the body of your dreams, but high-protein diets also cause a build-up of nitrogen in the body. Nitrogen is a breakdown product of protein, which is normally dealt with by the liver and kidneys and passed out of the body through the urine. But on a high-protein diet, excess nitrogen builds up and can damage the liver and kidneys.

Another mission in your quest to reduce fat around your middle is to control your body's natural inflammatory process. Unfortunately certain foods like red meat and dairy products produce substances called prostaglandins. These are not the healthy prostaglandins that can be created by essential fatty acids (see page 72). The particular prostaglandin produced from saturated fats is highly inflammatory. Called PGE2, this is produced from arachidonic acid (AA) (see diagram, page 73) of which one of the main sources is dairy products. For this reason, it would be better to use other forms of animal protein such as fish and eggs and reduce or eliminate dairy products from your diet. Of all the dairy products, organic, live, plain yogurt (not fruit yogurts as these can contain up to eight teaspoons of sugar) would be the best choice as it also contains beneficial bacteria that are helpful to the digestive system. Otherwise, use sheep's and goat's cheese rather than cow's and only in moderation.

AA is also present in red meat and although eggs contain AA they contain all the essential amino acids (hence they are called a 'first-class protein' or 'complete protein'). Research has shown that leucine, one of the essential amino acids found in eggs, can help with weight loss by stabilising blood sugar levels and encouraging the body to shed fat.[15]

And contrary to the old myth, although eggs are high in cholesterol they are low in saturated fats and can contain good amounts of Omega 3 essential fatty acids when the chickens have been fed well. Go for organic, free-range eggs (not just free-range) because the chicken's diet is extremely important to the quality of the eggs.

Try to ensure that you eat good-quality protein. I recommend fish (wild or organic, not farmed if you can), organic eggs, beans, nuts and seeds. I tend to advise avoiding red meat as it contains high levels of saturated fat and has been linked to both heart disease and bowel problems.

Reduce milk

There are many reasons why you should reduce milk in your diet:

- You might be lactose intolerant. This condition is estimated to affect 15 per cent of Caucasians and 70–90 per cent of Asians, black and American Indians because they stop producing the enzyme lactase which digests milk when they enter adulthood. Symptoms of lactose intolerance can range from minor digestive discomfort such as bloating and wind through to severe diarrhoea and abdominal pain. If you think you might be lactose intolerant try eliminating milk products from your diet for about a week to see if the symptoms disappear.
- The protein part of milk (casein) is also a known allergen and is often implicated in skin problems like eczema. Foods known to cause an allergic reaction such as milk or wheat (see page 62) do so by stimulating the adrenal glands. Most allergic reactions stimulate the release of histamine and other substances that produce inflammation. Cortisol is a strong anti-inflammatory so is called into play when there is an allergic reaction to a particular food. If you continue to eat foods which you suspect your body may be having difficulty dealing with, you will be boosting your cortisol levels and increasing your tendency to store fat. If you stop, the reaction changes. This is why people lose weight when they stop eating the foods they are reacting to. (For information on a test for food allergies see page 183.)
- A substance in milk, designed to give baby cows the best start in life, is thought to have a negative effect on human cells. Insulin-like Growth Factor (IGF-1), a substance that we produce naturally in our bodies, mainly in childhood, to encourage growth, is abundant in milk. The role of the growth factor is to support the growth and development of the young mammal for which that milk is designed. A calf has to be on its feet within hours of its birth and the emphasis for this animal is on physical development. Unfortunately IGF-1 is involved in cell multiplication and differentiation and research has shown that it acts as a strong mitogen (causing cells to divide) for a wide variety of cancer cell lines, including breast, prostate, lung and colon.[16]
- In 2005, a study in the *International Journal of Cancer* showed that drinking a glass of milk a day can increase a woman's risk of ovarian cancer.[17] It found an increased risk of up to 13 per cent connected to the milk sugar lactose. They showed no extra risk from yogurt or cheese and that is

because during the production of milk to make yogurt and cheese the fermentation process produces enzymes that break down lactose. So yogurt and cheese do not contain the milk sugar lactose.

- IGF-1 also prevents something called apoptosis (cell suicide – see page 41). This, as I explained in the previous chapter, is what happens with cancer. It could lead to the survival of cells that may be malignant. Even if the cancer warning isn't enough, as the name implies, IGF-1 has insulin-like properties in that it can stimulate the storage of glucose in fat cells.
- Increasing numbers of cows are fed antibiotics to speed up their growth and these drugs inevitably end up filtering through to us. There are major concerns that the overuse of antibiotics in general medicine will make certain illnesses like TB resistant to antibiotics and this is only made worse if we are exposed to antibiotics through our diet as well.
- The other problem is that cows have become milk machines as farmers try to get as much milk out of each one as possible. Whereas a generation ago, an individual cow would produce approximately 9 litres (2 gallons) of milk a day, today a cow can yield as many as 56 litres (12 gallons) a day. That is eight times more milk than any calf could drink. To produce that yield, milk production has to be stimulated unnaturally which must ultimately affect the milk.
- High temperatures used to pasteurise milk convert the fats in milk into trans fats (see page 75) which can increase the risk of heart disease.

All these factors knock milk products right down the list of 'ideal' foods.

Vegetarians

It used to be thought that vegetarians needed to combine a number of foods together in each meal in order to get all the eight essential amino acids. Now it is known that as long as a mixture of different foods is eaten over a day the body can obtain the eight essential amino acids from that day's intake. So a mixture of legumes, nuts, seeds and grains needs to be eaten over the day.

Soya is classed as a complete protein as it contains all the essential amino acids. However, I would only recommend using organic soya foods because any other could be genetically modified. It is also best to eat soya as it is traditionally eaten by other cultures, such as the Japanese, in the form of tofu, miso, soya sauce (tamari is wheat free) and tempeh.

Avoid any soya products made from soya protein isolate (check ingredients labels) as the process used to produce these results in a 'food' that not only no longer resembles the original soya bean but also contains traces of aluminium and nitrates. Up to 60 per cent of processed foods contain soya (e.g. bread, biscuits, pizza and baby food) and in the majority of cases this takes the form of soya isolate and is not derived from whole soya beans. The best way to tell a whole soya product from a soya isolate product is to look at the ingredients list. Also, at the moment, if a food is labelled organic it is not genetically modified.

Another good protein source for vegetarians is quinoa, which is actually a seed but is used as a grain. It is high in protein and rich in vitamins and minerals.

Seaweed is a good food for vegetarians and non-vegetarians alike – it is low in calories and has a very good mineral content including zinc, manganese, chromium, selenium, calcium, magnesium, iron and especially iodine. Iodine is essential for the healthy functioning of the thyroid gland which regulates metabolism. Different types of seaweed include nori, kombu (Japanese equivalent of kelp), agar, arame and hiziki.

6. Eat essential fats

Whilst many people believe that 'fat makes you fat', you should by now understand that the real culprits are sugar and refined carbohydrates in foods and drink. These increase the production of insulin (the fat-storing hormone) and then the release of the stress hormones that make you fat.

Research from Harvard School of Public Health has confirmed that reducing fat is not the answer to losing weight. Dr Walter Willett has stated that 'diets high in fat do not appear to be the primary cause of the high prevalence of excess body fat in our society'[18] and that 'the emphasis on total fat reduction has been a serious distraction in efforts to control obesity and improve health in general.'[19] The research suggests that all the emphasis on low-fat foods has been a red herring, borne out by the fact that (particularly in the USA) over the last two decades there has been a substantial decline in fat consumption and a corresponding massive increase in obesity.

Bad fats

Bad – saturated – fats are found in red meat and dairy products. There is no doubt that saturated fats are not good for your general health as they can increase the risk of heart disease and bowel cancer. They also increase the risk of insulin resistance because they make the cell membranes hard and less receptive to insulin. However, the most lethal combination is to put them together with refined carbohydrates and sugar (your classic takeaway burger meal with the white bun). They will increase both cholesterol and triglycerides (fats in the blood) and therefore the risk of both heart attacks and strokes.

Good fats

A lifelong dependency on low-fat diets might mean that you consume fewer saturated fats, but at the same time you will be making yourself deficient in the unsaturated fats, also known as essential fatty acids (EFAs). As their name implies, EFAs (found in nuts, seeds and oily fish) are essential and can only be obtained from your diet as your body cannot manufacture them.

An EFA deficiency can cause any of the following:

- difficulty in losing weight
- dry skin
- cracked skin on heels or fingertips
- hair loss
- lifeless hair
- poor wound healing
- dandruff
- depression
- irritability
- soft or brittle nails
- allergies
- dry eyes
- lack of motivation
- aching joints
- fatigue
- high blood pressure
- arthritis
- premenstrual syndrome (PMS)
- painful breasts

Many of the women I see in my clinic experience the symptoms above and confess that they do not eat nuts, seeds, oily fish or avocados. Why? Because they think they are fattening. And yet they find that they can't lose weight and end up with raging deficiency symptoms!

Essential fats are essential because:

- they slow down the rate at which the stomach empties, so making carbohydrates even more slow-releasing
- they boost your metabolism
- they make you less insulin resistant
- they reduce inflammation

When fat is added to a carbohydrate it works in the same way as adding protein, slowing down the rate at which food enters the intestines. So by adding fat (unsaturated of course) to a carbohydrate you improve its value to your diet. This can be as simple as adding nuts and seeds to porridge for breakfast (nuts and seeds are doubly helpful as they contain both protein and essential fats). Or you could drizzle good-quality, cold-pressed organic sesame or sunflower oil or extra virgin olive oil over roasted vegetables just before you serve them.

Essential fats really can help you to lose weight because they boost your metabolism. The Omega 3 EFAs specifically help with fat burning because they direct blood sugar towards the glycogen stores to be burned as fuel instead of being stored as fat. They also help to increase fat and cholesterol metabolism meaning that less is available to clog up your arteries. In the year 2000 the US Nurses' Health Study involving 85,000 women found that the risk of heart attack in those who ate fish containing these EFAs just once a week was 29 per cent lower than in those who ate it less than once a month. Women who ate it five times a week have half the risk of dying of a heart attack.[20]

So EFAs help to budge fat around the middle by reversing insulin resistance. That is why EFAs also curb depression because they help brain cells to be more fluid so neurotransmitters can then do their job properly.

The EFAs also help to reduce inflammation by controlling prostaglandin production (see page 67). This is important because, as I explained earlier, excess weight around the middle leads to low-grade inflammation which hampers the body's ability to use insulin.

Your body uses EFAs to produce substances called prostaglandins (hormone-like substances). These prostaglandins help to prevent inflammation, regulate the immune system and reduce abnormal blood clotting.

Unfortunately, your body can also produce 'bad' prostaglandins which cause inflammation.

PGE2 is classed as a 'bad' prostaglandin because it increases inflammation and blood clotting. PGE1 and PGE3 are classed as 'good' prostaglandins as they are anti-inflammatory, prevent blood clots and lower blood pressure.

From the diagram on page 73, you can see that the Omega 3 series of EFAs (alpha-linolenic acid) found in oily fish, linseeds (flaxseeds), walnuts, soya, pumpkin seeds and green leafy vegetables are converted into the good prostaglandin PGE3.

But the Omega 6 series of EFAs (linoleic acid) found in nuts and seeds can be converted to either 'good' PGE1 or 'bad' PGE2 prostaglandins.

When you have high levels of insulin your body tends to stop the conversion of the Omega 6 EFAs into PGE1 and instead produces more of the 'bad' PGE2. So this increases inflammation which, in turn, stops your body responding to insulin. This then causes more inflammation. Round and round it goes, with more and more weight piling on your middle.

• HOW OMEGA 3 EFAS FIGHT INSULIN RESISTANCE •

Omega 3 EFAs are crucial for the correct functioning of cell membranes, which are made up of 60 per cent fat. They help the membranes to be more fluid and flexible and this results in the receptors on the cells being more sensitive to insulin. Insulin receptors are on the outer part of the cell that allows the cell to bind or join with insulin that is in the blood. When the cell and insulin bind together the cell can take glucose from the blood and use it for energy.

Essential Fatty Acids

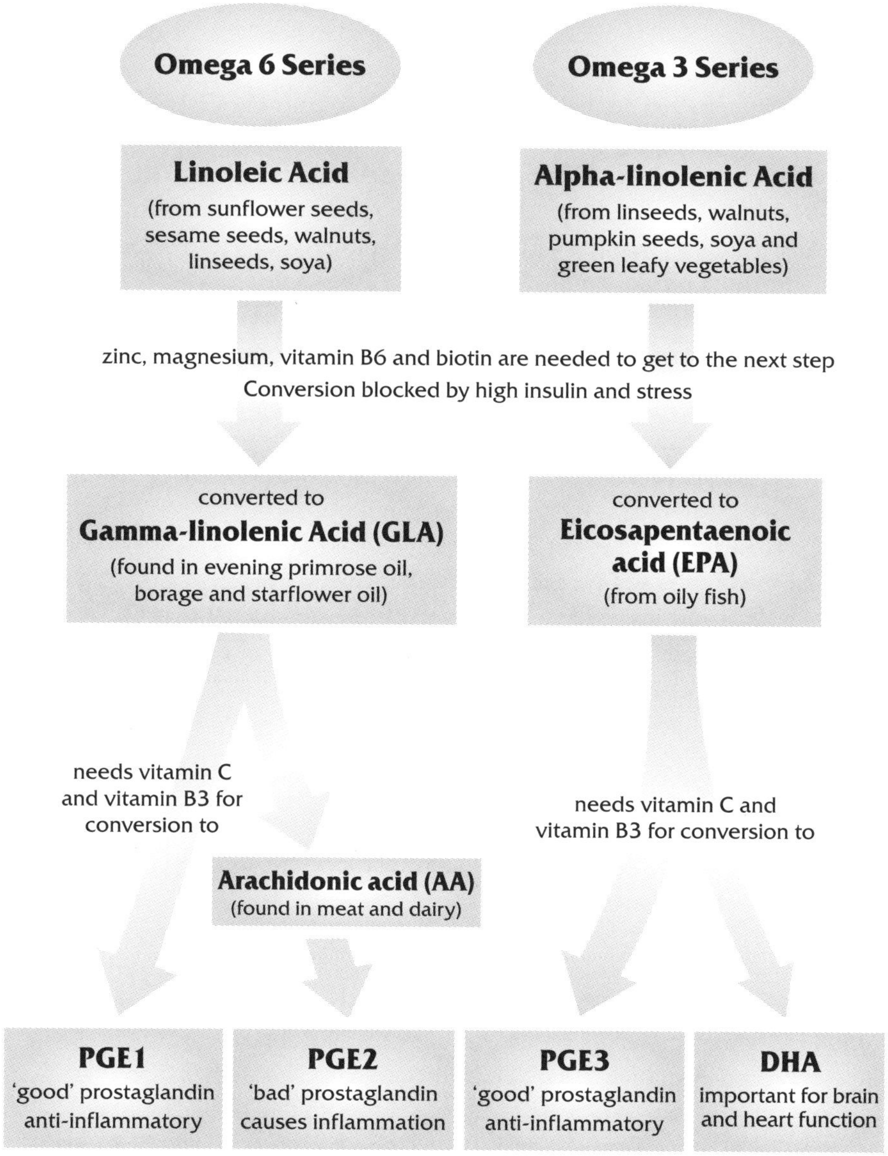

Omega 6 Series

Linoleic Acid
(from sunflower seeds, sesame seeds, walnuts, linseeds, soya)

Omega 3 Series

Alpha-linolenic Acid
(from linseeds, walnuts, pumpkin seeds, soya and green leafy vegetables)

zinc, magnesium, vitamin B6 and biotin are needed to get to the next step
Conversion blocked by high insulin and stress

converted to
Gamma-linolenic Acid (GLA)
(found in evening primrose oil, borage and starflower oil)

converted to
Eicosapentaenoic acid (EPA)
(from oily fish)

needs vitamin C and vitamin B3 for conversion to

Arachidonic acid (AA)
(found in meat and dairy)

needs vitamin C and vitamin B3 for conversion to

PGE1	PGE2	PGE3	DHA
'good' prostaglandin anti-inflammatory	'bad' prostaglandin causes inflammation	'good' prostaglandin anti-inflammatory	important for brain and heart function

Breaking this vicious circle can be done in a number of ways. For best effect, they should all be undertaken at the same time:

- As you can see from the diagram, your body uses an enzyme to convert Omega 6 EFAs to GLA and Omega 3 to EPA and DHA but this conversion gets blocked by stress hormones and insulin. So you need to work on controlling stress (see Chapter 7).

- Your body needs vitamin B6, magnesium, zinc and biotin to make this conversion so for a while these should be added to the diet as supplements (see Chapter 5). The more stressed you are, the more your body calls on supplies of different vitamins and minerals and the more deficient you become the more you make it impossible to convert the EFAs efficiently.
- High levels of insulin will cause the Omega 6 oils to be converted into arachidonic acid (AA) which produces the 'bad' prostaglandin PGE2. If you follow the recommendations in this book you'll be doing the best you can to reduce insulin so that less of the Omega 6 oils are converted to the 'bad' inflammatory prostaglandins.
- If you increase your consumption of Omega 3 this not only produces PGE3, the anti-inflammatory prostaglandins, but also blocks the conversion of Omega 6 EFAs to AA.

There's no point taking GLA supplements (evening primrose oil or starflower oil for example) if your insulin levels are high, as the GLA is converted into AA and then into PGE2 – the 'bad' prostaglandin.

Years ago we all used to get a good balance of Omega 3 and Omega 6 oils from our food but now a typical Western diet contains nearly ten times more Omega 6 (from the increased use of vegetable oils and seeds) than Omega 3 (oily fish, soya, linseeds) resulting in much higher levels of these 'bad' inflammatory prostaglandins in our normal diets.

I would recommend a three-month push of boosting your Omega 3 intake in supplement form (see Chapter 5) to kick-start your fat-burning mechanism. As the stress hormones will block the conversion of Omega 3 to EPA it is better to take the supplements as EPA rather than as fish oil or Omega 3 so that this bypasses any problems and you automatically produce the 'good' prostaglandins PGE3.

Vegetarians who eat no fish but who are fat around the middle will find this a bit more difficult because the stress hormones will block the conversion of Omega 3 oils in linseeds (flax), soya and walnuts to EPA. So it is important to follow the recommendations in this book to control your cortisol levels. Research has shown that if you reduce the amount of Omega 6 vegetable oils in your diet, the conversion rate of Omega 3 to EPA will be higher.[21] So concentrate on using nuts and seeds, which give both protein and EFAs, rather than trying to get your EFAs from vegetable oils.

What about olive oil?

Olive oil is not classed as an essential fatty acid. It is an Omega 9 monounsaturated fat. Olive oil is high in monounsaturated fat and has been found to lower LDL ('bad' cholesterol) and raise HDL ('good' cholesterol). This is one of the factors that contribute to the low rate of heart disease in the

Mediterranean where olive oil is a staple. To achieve a better balance between Omega 6 and Omega 3 EFAs, I would suggest sticking to olive oil rather than using an Omega 6 EFA like sunflower oil.

Taking care of your cooking oils

If you overheat oil, leave it in direct sunlight or re-use it after cooking it can quickly oxidise, leaving it open to attack by highly reactive chemical fragments called free radicals. These have been linked to cancer, coronary heart disease, rheumatoid arthritis and premature ageing. Free radicals speed up the ageing process by destroying healthy cells as well attacking collagen (the 'cement' that holds cells together).

To prevent this from happening, choose cold-pressed, unrefined vegetable oils or extra virgin olive oil. Unfortunately most standard supermarket oils are manufactured using chemicals and heat to extract as much oil as possible from each batch. This ruins the nutritional content and quality of the oil. Choose organic oil if you can and store it away from light.

Avoid frying with polyunsaturated fats such as sunflower oil as they become unstable when heated. Use olive oil or butter for frying. Monounsaturated olive oil is less likely to cause free radicals and butter does not because it is a saturated fat. Keep cooking temperatures as low as possible and bake, steam, roast or grill instead of frying as much as you can.

Trans fats – the big fat villains

If saturated fats are bad, trans fats are even worse. They are made by taking a polyunsaturated oil like sunflower oil and passing hydrogen through it at a high temperature and pressure. This changes the molecular structure of the oil making it more solid and spreadable (for margarine) and giving it a much longer shelf life. You'll find trans fats (labelled hydrogenated vegetable oil) in all sorts of convenience foods, cakes and biscuits – pretty much all processed food.

Trans fats, once eaten, end up like plastic in your gut which your body really struggles to deal with. They stop the absorption of essential fats from your diet and increase the risk of a heart attack. One study showed that the HDL ('good' cholesterol) levels in people on a trans-fat diet were 21 per cent lower than those on a saturated-fat diet. And just by increasing their consumption of trans fats by 2 per cent they elevated their risk of heart disease by a massive 30 per cent.[22] Trans fats also increase the 'bad' cholesterol (LDL) and, interestingly, as the dietary intake of trans fats increased the LDL molecules got smaller. This is very negative (see page 34) as the molecules stick to the walls of the arteries as plaque (called atherosclerosis).[23]

Trans fats can also increase the chances of becoming insulin resistant as they harden cell membranes making them less receptive to insulin. They have now been linked to increasing the risk of Type 2 diabetes.[24]

So always check labels. 'Made from sunflower oil' on a margarine tub can mean that through the hydrogenation process the oil will have changed into something quite unrecognisable. I would recommend using either organic butter in moderation or unhydrogenated margarine (available in health food shops), rather than ordinary margarine. Always read the labels and look at the ingredient list and steer well clear of any mention of hydrogenated fats or oils.

In 2004 the Danish government ruled that oils and fats containing more than 2 per cent trans fats should no longer be sold in Denmark. It would be good if other countries followed suit.

7. Don't eat on the run

To be truly committed to this programme you will need to control the cortisol that is putting the weight around your middle. You need to keep your blood sugar in balance, which in turn stops the production of the stress hormones, and make it clear to your body that you are not under stress by following the recommendations in Chapter 7. Your body does not care what triggers the stress response – be it internal (blood sugar swings) or external (traffic jam); the response and the weight gain around the middle will be the same.

If you persistently eat on the run you will be giving your body the message that time is scarce, that you are under pressure and that you are stressed. We know that if you eat under stress your digestive system shuts down because your body prefers to reserve its energy and resources for saving your life and not for digesting that sandwich (see page 13). As a result, you could end up feeling bloated and uncomfortable after eating because the food could be just sitting there fermenting in your gut.

The idea is to give your body a different message. Tell it that you are not under attack, that all is calm. Only then can your digestive system do its job properly and absorb all the vital vitamins and minerals from your food.

In order to achieve this you must make a point of sitting down and eating your meals in as calm a way as possible. Even if you can only manage ten minutes, make sure that you sit down, chew well, calm your mind and enjoy the food. Don't just shovel it in. Snacks may be eaten on the run if necessary as they normally involve a much smaller amount of food, and it is preferable to have a snack within three hours of a meal (to avoid a blood sugar drop) rather than not have it at all.

Chewing well is important because the first part of digestion takes place in your mouth. It also signals to the other parts of your digestive system that they should get ready to receive food. So if you do not chew well, the first part of breakdown in the mouth does not happen, your digestive system does not get the signal to prepare itself and your food will drop down to your stomach in larger molecules than it can really manage.

Another advantage of eating slowly is you are less likely to overeat. Once you start eating it takes twenty minutes for your brain to register that you are full. So if you eat slowly you will end up eating less food because your brain will tell you that you have had enough. If you eat quickly you can consume a lot more food than you actually need before your brain registers this. There is a big difference between hunger and appetite.

Remember also that you should not drink whilst you are eating.

8. Watch what you drink

You need to control cortisol by restricting foods that cause a fast release of blood sugar, but what you drink is important too.

Caffeine

Coffee, black tea, green tea, chocolate, colas and other soft drinks and some medications such as headache remedies all contain caffeine. And although many people do not realise it, tea and coffee are not only fattening, they also specifically cause fat to be deposited around your middle.

Caffeine is a stimulant which prompts your body to release cortisol which in turn triggers the release of insulin. Over time caffeine will make your body resistant to insulin so that it turns glucose straight into fat and stores it around your middle. In research it was estimated that caffeine decreases insulin sensitivity by 15 per cent in people without diabetes.[25] Caffeine also increased the levels of free 'bad' fatty acids in the blood and also levels of the hormone adrenaline. The researchers estimated that the decrease in insulin sensitivity caused by the caffeine matched the increase in insulin sensitivity from taking insulin-sensitising drugs like Metformin. So people who are on insulin-sensitising medication might not need this medication if they eliminated caffeine. But it can also mean that the caffeine can be cancelling out the effect of drugs.[26] (**Note**: do not stop any medication without consulting your doctor.) One study even went so far as to be entitled 'Caffeine: a cause of insulin resistance?'[27] so in order to shift that weight around the middle caffeine needs to go.

Drinking caffeinated beverages is yet another way of telling your body that it is under attack and must store fat. To convince your body that it is allowed to let go of this stored fat, you need to eliminate caffeine from your diet.

To your body, drinking caffeinated drinks is equivalent to doing something stressful. When researchers compared men given the caffeine equivalent of two to three cups of coffee with men doing stressful tasks, they found that the caffeine raised the stress hormones (like cortisol) to the same level as that found in the men who were doing the stressful tasks.[28]

Another problem is that caffeine is addictive. Tea and coffee act like a drug: as the effects of the caffeine begin to wear off, you will want more and then you will be back on that rollercoaster again (see page 51). It's a classic crutch for that mid-afternoon energy dip when you feel that you'll never make it without a cup of coffee and a biscuit. And if you add sugar to your tea or coffee the rollercoaster highs will be higher and the lows lower, causing even more damage to your body.

Caffeine is fast acting and very permeable which means that it passes easily through the blood-brain barrier. It has been suggested that 'within an hour of drinking a cup of coffee there is probably caffeine in every cell of your body and traces to be found in all your body fluids.'[29] Caffeine works by blocking the neurotransmitter adenosine, associated with depression, inhibition of gastric section, slowing of the heartbeat and general lowering of neural activity.[30] So caffeine increases the heart rate, blood pressure and gastric activity. It has also been shown to increase another neurotransmitter, dopamine, which is how the stimulants amphetamine and cocaine work.[31]

Because caffeine acts like a drug, you should not attempt to eliminate it suddenly from your diet and go 'cold turkey' as this could cause quite dramatic withdrawal symptoms such as headaches, nausea, tiredness, muscle cramps and depression. To minimise these effects, you should try cutting down gradually over a period of a few weeks. Start by substituting decaffeinated coffee for half of your total coffee intake each day and gradually switch over completely to decaffeinated. Then, slowly substitute other drinks, such as herbal teas and grain coffees. Your ultimate aim, ideally, should be to do away with decaffeinated coffee as well because it still contains other stimulants (theobromine and theophylline) that are not removed when the coffee is decaffeinated.

Cola is just as bad. Many women are hopelessly addicted – I've seen women who drink as many as eight cans a day. Because colas are often a combination of caffeine and artificial sweeteners they should also be removed from your diet, but, again, this should be done slowly, perhaps at a rate of one can a day.

And chocolate is no innocent either – it also contains the dastardly caffeine. And it's no good switching to organic, dark chocolate; although it has less sugar, its percentage of cocoa solids is higher than in milk chocolate, making the caffeine effect even stronger.

You will know when your body is starting to get the 'let go of fat' message because that urge for a cup of coffee or tea will have disappeared. Once you have managed four clear caffeine-free weeks you could start to add a supplement of green tea (see Chapter 5). Green tea (which is made from unfermented leaves) does contain caffeine but it also has high levels of antioxidants called polyphenols. These have been found to have anti-cancer properties[32] and also help to reduce cholesterol and increase HDL – 'good' cholesterol.[33] Polyphenols have also been studied for their effect on weight and body fat and a twelve-week trial using green tea extract showed a significant reduction in waist circumference, BMI and percentage body fat.[34] So whilst I would not recommend drinking green tea for three months after cutting out caffeine, it is fine to take it in supplement form to help with fat loss as the supplement contains very little caffeine.

Alcohol

Think of the classic 'beer' belly and you have the apple shape in dramatic action. Quite simply, beer (a liquid carbohydrate) hits the bloodstream quickly, causing the release of cortisol and insulin and, eventually, insulin resistance. So if you want to shift that weight around the middle you will need to eliminate alcohol for a few weeks. If you absolutely can't resist a drop of something, remember that wine has less of an effect than beer, and spirits have the least effect of all.

Alcohol is harmful in a number of other ways. It acts as an anti-nutrient, meaning that it blocks the good effects of your food by depleting the body of vitamins and minerals, especially zinc, calcium, magnesium, vitamin C and also the B vitamins. These vitamins and minerals, especially the B vitamins (known as the 'stress' vitamins) are vital in helping your body to cope with stress, as you will see in the next chapter.

Alcohol also interferes with the metabolism of the EFAs needed to produce the 'good' prostaglandins (see page 70) that control inflammation.

Alcohol acts as a diuretic (as does coffee), making you lose water and feel dehydrated. The body typically registers this as a stress (as it would with a famine) and so raises cortisol levels.

Your liver is the waste disposal and detoxifying unit of the body, not only for alcohol but also for toxins, waste products, drugs and the hormones your body produces. The liver is the largest organ in your body and has many other functions such as fat metabolism (absorption, emulsification, transport and storage), production of bile, protein metabolism, cholesterol production, manufacture of fibrinogen (a substance that helps the blood to clot), production of enzymes and of course blood sugar control. So the last thing you should do is compromise your liver function by plying it with alcohol whilst it has so much other work to do. Add the effects of chronic stress because it thinks your life is in danger and you can see that the liver can become so overloaded that it is not really doing the job it was designed to do.

Another concern is that cholesterol is produced by your liver and cholesterol is the starting block for the manufacture of the stress hormones. So, if your liver registers that you are under constant stress from either the blood sugar rollercoaster or pressure of work, it will produce yet more cholesterol.

My advice, therefore, is for you to give your liver a rest for at least four weeks by cutting out all alcohol and following the supplement and herb recommendations in the next chapter to boost liver function. If you really feel you have to drink alcohol – say at a big function or family celebration – make sure you only do so on a full stomach and with a meal that contains some fats or oils to slow the absorption of the alcohol. This is actually a good tip for whenever you drink alcohol generally speaking. A 'liquid lunch' is never a good idea.

Soft drinks

Soft drinks often contain high-fructose corn syrup and their increased consumption has been linked with the rise in obesity seen in the USA.[35] These drinks are effectively liquid sugar and, as such, are rapidly absorbed into the bloodstream, kicking off the blood sugar rollercoaster and the storage of fat. Furthermore, it is not helpful to substitute soft drinks that contain artificial sweeteners instead of high-fructose corn syrup, because these can also increase your appetite and have been associated with other health problems – see page 65).

The concern is greatest for children and teenagers whose schools can be given up to £12,000 in 'grants' to install soft drink vending machines on the school premises. We are now seeing children as young as eleven and twelve with fat around the middle and Type 2 diabetes. The American soft drink culture has a lot to answer for.

Fruit juice

When you're trying to combat the fat stored around your middle you need to be wary of fruit juice. As discussed on page 62, it hits the bloodstream fairly quickly because it is concentrated fruit sugar without any fibre. I recommend avoiding it completely for at least the first four weeks, then reintroducing it in dilute form – half water–half juice. You might like to try it with sparkling water to make it a little bit more interesting. Always drink juice with a snack to slow down its absorption.

Also, read the labels on juice cartons. If it says 'fruit drink' then you know that it will not be pure fruit. Many fruit drinks contain as little as 5 per cent fruit, the other 95 per cent being sugar, colourings, sweeteners and water.

Water

Water is absolutely essential for every function of the body. It is needed for digestion, absorption, circulation and excretion. Whilst we might survive without food for five weeks we cannot live for more than five days without water. Our bodies are made up of more than 70 per cent water and every drop of that is needed to help transport nutrients and waste products in and out of the cells, carry waste out of the body and maintain body temperature.

Most of us do not drink enough water – we should all drink at least six glasses a day. Try hot water and a slice of lemon before breakfast: it's

Your guide to Bottled Water

Navigating your way through the maze of bottled waters in the supermarket can be confusing, so here is a quick guide:

Spring water is usually taken from one or more underground sources and has undergone a range of treatments, such as filtration and blending.

Natural mineral water is bottled in its natural underground state and is untreated. It has to come from an officially registered source, conform to purity standards and carry details of its source and mineral analysis on its label.

Naturally sparkling water is natural water from an underground source with enough naturally occurring carbon dioxide to make it bubbly.

Sparkling (carbonated) water has had carbon dioxide added during bottling just as ordinary fizzy drinks do.

Watch out for flavoured spring waters as whilst they sound wonderfully natural, they often contain sugar or artificial sweeteners and other 'nasties'. And it is better to buy water in glass bottles as plastic can contaminate the water with xenoestrogens.

In my opinion, therefore, the best option is to drink still mineral water in glass bottles.

wonderfully refreshing and excellent for the liver. Herbal teas do count towards your liquid intake but other drinks don't.

Tap water is not ideal because in many areas it is contaminated with arsenic, lead or copper from pipes. Other substances such as pesticides and fertilisers can also leach into the water through the ground. Filtering water (either in a jug, or with a device plumbed under your sink) helps, but will not eliminate every impurity. Some filters can also help to filter out xenoestrogens (foreign oestrogens).

9. Change the way in which you think about food

This section is about changing the way in which you think about food and eating. The word 'diet' has temporary connotations, implying that it will be short lived, and this is not what I am advocating. If you are really serious about changing your body shape you need to start thinking about food and eating in terms of your lifestyle so that healthy, enjoyable eating becomes a habit, something you do every day without a thought.

But you don't have to be a total mung bean eater, or at least not all the time. Aim to eat well 80 per cent of the time to get rid of that fat around the middle and give yourself 20 per cent leeway.

Many of the women I see in my clinic talk about having been 'good' or 'bad' as far as eating is concerned. However, thinking like this will only make you

• OLD HABITS •

Contrary to what you may have been told as a child, you do not have to finish everything on your plate. Turn the old habit around. Each time you eat, try to make a habit of leaving something on your plate and over time you will realise that you are eating less without even thinking about it.

Also you do not need to eat your children's leftovers, especially if they are eating at around five or six o'clock in the evening and you will be eating your dinner at eight.

feel guilty and is self-defeating. Keep your aims in mind and focus on the positive. Talk to yourself in positive terms – the mind believes what it hears. So comments like 'I am never going to lose this belly' can become a self-fulfilling prophecy. Talk instead about 'liking yourself' and look forward to 'being able to wear that skirt again'.

Why bother?

After just a few weeks on my plan you will look and feel better. You will have started to lose the apple shape that's been dogging you for years, and you will also be feeling more energetic and healthy. You will have set yourself up to be healthier in the future with a good chance of preventing serious illnesses later on.

In 2004 a report called 'Storing Up Problems: the Medical Case for a Slimmer Nation' was launched in the UK by three major medical bodies (the Royal College of Physicians, the Faculty of Public Health and the Royal College of Paediatrics and Child Health). Together, they called for a national strategy to halt obesity and put a stop to the frightening inevitability that within the next fifteen years one in three adults will be obese. They highlighted the following:

- Obesity in women between 1980 and 2002 went up threefold from 8 to 23 per cent.
- English teenagers are the fattest in Europe.
- One in four young English children between the ages of thirteen and seventeen is obese or overweight (as highlighted at the European Congress in Obesity in 2005).
- England has one of the biggest weight problems for seven- to eleven-year-olds with 27 per cent of them being obese or overweight.

The Congress also revealed that 60,000 overweight British children, some as young as eleven have the metabolic syndrome (Syndrome X – see page 30).

We live in a time when degenerative diseases have become epidemics. Illnesses such as cancer, coronary heart disease, stroke, diabetes, arthritis and auto-immune conditions are on the increase, and they are the cause of death and disability in a huge percentage of the population. In the West very few of us die of 'old age'. We are dying of diseases that take time to manifest themselves in our bodies. They are not a 'natural' part of ageing, but the result of the appalling way in which many of us treat our bodies over the years. For example, arthritis is a common feature of old age in the West whereas in other cultures it simply does not exist to the same degree. Does the fact that it is common make it acceptable? I think not.

A massive study of 85,000 nurses in the USA which started in 1976 has shown the enormous difference a healthy lifestyle can make. It has shown that a whopping 83 per cent of heart disease problems could be prevented just by keeping the following five 'rules':[36]

- not smoking
- maintaining a normal weight (BMI of less than 25)
- taking moderate exercise (more than thirty minutes a day)
- drinking no more than two alcoholic drinks a day
- eating a good diet low in trans fats, with a higher ratio of polyunsaturated fat to saturated fat, high in fibre, high in fish and high in folic acid

I would agree with all these rules with the exception that for my plan to really work, you need to set alcohol consumption at zero for a while.

The researchers of this study also looked at the risk of Type 2 diabetes and came up with the astonishing conclusion that 'a healthy lifestyle can prevent most cases of Type 2 diabetes'.[37]

Research like this really shows that illnesses like cancer, coronary heart disease, stroke and diabetes (the spokes of that wheel on page 37) are not 'just one of those things'. They are preventable even if you have a high family history risk. It is up to you to make the changes in your diet and lifestyle – no one else will do it for you.

You have to make the decision to take responsibility for your health. However, this does not mean allowing a drug to control problems such as high blood sugar or cholesterol. The drug may alleviate symptoms, but will not address the cause of why your body is producing too much cholesterol, for example.

The fact that you are reading this book is a good sign. It means that you are beginning to take responsibility by searching for answers other than drugs. But be warned: there is no quick fix for losing that fat around the middle or for staying healthy either.

Having said that, with a little effort and a positive mindset you can achieve your aims in just three months. You will need to look closely at your diet and also your lifestyle in general (see Chapter 7). And there are some specific vitamins, minerals and herbs that can make the whole 'lose-your-belly' process faster and easier, as you will read in the next chapter.

• Chapter 5 •

SUPPLEMENTS TO HELP CHANGE YOUR SHAPE

Vitamins, minerals and herbs that will enable you to lose that bulge

If you store fat around your middle, the chances are that yours is not a recently developed problem. Most apple-shaped people have been unconsciously exacerbating their unhealthy body shape for quite some time.

To turn things around effectively there is no doubt that you need to halt your body's rollercoaster of blood sugar swings (see page 51) by making the dietary changes recommended in Chapter 4. And these measures must be taken in tandem with the lifestyle recommendations in Chapter 7. However, in most cases, because your body has been under constant stress for so long it is likely that it will need a bit of extra support and encouragement to accept that it is safe to burn off that fat and restore you to good health. That takes time – around three months – as your body needs to adapt gradually for the effects to be permanent.

Whilst some sectors of the medical establishment are sceptical about supplements, there are plenty of medical studies endorsing them and I have seen dramatic results with my own eyes. I have treated women suffering with many problems, for example tachycardia (in which the heart beats frighteningly fast). They were referred by their GPs to a cardiologist for standard heart checks to rule out anything serious and, in each case, they were sent home with the 'all clear' and continuing symptoms. It was clear to me that something had to be causing their hearts to beat faster. So, once I was happy that there was nothing wrong with their actual heart function, I suggested a programme to control stress hormones, through healthy eating (as described in Chapter 4), adapting lifestyle factors that might have been causing them stress, and a programme of supplements and herbs aimed specifically at calming down the adrenal function. Within three months their symptoms had gone.

Research has shown that certain vitamins, minerals, essential fatty acids (EFAs), herbs and other nutrients can help you to lose that apple shape more quickly than you would with just changes in your diet alone. And once you have lost the fat around the middle you can switch to a simple maintenance programme of supplements (see Chapter 11).

Below are listed all the supplements and herbs that can and do make a difference in helping you to lose that fat around the middle, together with the reasons why and how they work. It is an extensive list but this does not mean that you will need to go out and buy all the supplements individually as many of them are combined in one supplement. (For a more concise guide to what supplements to take see Chapter 10.)

WHY SUPPLEMENT?

Because your body has been pumping out high levels of adrenaline and cortisol over extended periods of time, it will have had to call on supplies of vitamins and minerals to deal with this. This means that the longer you are stressed, the more nutritionally deficient your body becomes. It is mainly vitamin C, the B vitamins, magnesium and zinc that are affected, so it's important to take these in supplement form for three months to correct any basic deficiencies.

A number of chemical reactions are involved in turning glucose into energy (the good reaction) instead of fat (the bad reaction). These are controlled by enzymes, which are themselves dependent on certain vitamins and minerals in the body. If you're low on these nutrients, your body will find it harder to let go of that weight. You are also very likely to be deficient in a number of vitamins and minerals if you, like so many other women, have been yo-yo dieting for many years, either restricting food intake or using different diet drinks or pills.

There is a strong and frequently repeated argument that we should be able to get all the nutrients we need from a well-balanced diet and yes, in theory we should. The problem is, however, that all too often we can't. Food that is rich in nutrients needs to be grown in soil that is rich in nutrients, but much of our soil has been over-farmed to the point that it no longer contains the nutrients we need. Pesticides and other chemicals reduce the nutrient content of our food, and processing strips our food of its key nutrients further still. Chemicals in processed food put an additional strain on our bodies, increasing our need for key nutrients even more.

WHAT CAN SUPPLEMENTS DO?

Supplements have the ability to:

- make your body less insulin resistant, or in other words more insulin *sensitive* so that it is able to use effectively the insulin that you produce help your body to remove glucose from the blood
- calm your adrenal glands so that they produce the correct level of hormones
- help your body to burn off excess fat

So nowadays it is not that easy to get everything you need from your diet. A *Which?* report in 2005 found, for instance, that one pack of sliced green beans contained only 11 per cent of the vitamin C it should have had. And a recent national study showed that 74 per cent of women were falling woefully short on nutrients in their diet. The National Diet and Nutritional survey published in 2003 which looked at adults aged between nineteen and sixty-four showed that only 15 per cent of women and 13 per cent of men actually achieved the five-a-day target for fruit and vegetables. Seventy-four per cent of women failed to achieve the reference nutrient intake (RNI – this term has replaced the old RDA, recommended daily allowance) for magnesium, 45 per cent for zinc, 84 per cent for folic acid and 15 per cent for vitamin D.

MIGHTY MINERALS

Chromium

What does it do?

One of the most important minerals in this 'lose-your-belly' plan, chromium is needed for the metabolism of sugar. It helps insulin to take glucose into the cells; without chromium, insulin is less effective at controlling blood sugar levels and glucose levels rise.

Few people have enough chromium in their diet. The mineral should be naturally present in grains such as oats, rice, wheat, corn and rye. However, as soon as these grains are refined (turned into white bread, pastries, biscuits and even pasta) the chromium is stripped out. It's yet another vicious circle: chromium is vital to keep blood sugar in balance, but is not present in refined foods. Yet refined food is part of the cause of the blood sugar imbalance. To make matters worse, if refined foods are eaten with sugar (as is often the case), chromium will be stripped from the body through urine and sweat.

Chromium plays a major role in weight control. It is the most widely researched mineral used in the treatment of obesity partly because it helps to control cravings and reduces hunger. One study showed that people who took chromium over a ten-week period lost an average of 1.9kg (4.2lb) of fat whilst those on a placebo (dummy tablet) lost only 0.2kg (0.4lb).[1]

Chromium helps your body to reverse insulin resistance by allowing cells to become more sensitive to insulin once more and it's been found that people with the lowest levels of chromium tend to have the most problems with glucose and insulin regulation.[2] Chromium has also been found to help in breaking down fat and cholesterol in the blood, and deficiency has not only been linked to high blood glucose but also high cholesterol and the development of plaque in the arteries.[3] People with Type 2 diabetes tend to have lower levels of chromium[4] so it is thought that a chromium deficiency may play a major part in the increasing problem of hypoglycaemia, diabetes and obesity.[5]

Chromium has also been shown to reduce levels of the stress hormone, cortisol. This was tested on cattle and sheep that produced high levels of cortisol from the stress of being transported over long distances.[6]

Best form to take

I recommend taking chromium in the form of polynicotinate which is a yeast-free form bound to niacin (vitamin B3). I suggest avoiding chromium in the form of picolinate as this is a synthetic form and there have been concerns that chromium picolinate might be linked to DNA damage, liver dysfunction, skin blisters and anaemia.[7] Chromium polynicotinate does not cause any of these problems and as one study says, 'Niacin-bound chromium has been demonstrated to be more bioavailable and efficacious and no toxicity has been reported.'[8]

WARNING

Consult your doctor before taking a chromium supplement if you are diabetic and on medication.

Magnesium

What does it do?

Known as 'Nature's tranquilliser', magnesium calms the adrenal glands and helps to balance blood sugar by contributing to the production and action of insulin. Diabetics are often deficient in magnesium.[9]

The higher your magnesium levels the greater your sensitivity to insulin (which is a good thing) and there is a strong link between magnesium deficiency and insulin resistance.[10] A study of 12,000 people over six years showed that people with the lowest intake of magnesium had a 94 per cent chance of developing Type 2 diabetes.[11]

Magnesium levels tend to be depleted when you're under stress, so if you have fat around the middle and high cortisol levels, the chances are you'll be lacking in magnesium. I see a lot of women in the clinic who are worried about their calcium levels, especially around the menopause, but in fact, when tested, the majority are found to be low in magnesium, not calcium.

Magnesium is important not only for insulin production, but also for its involvement in energy production, bone health, blood clotting, muscle relaxation and regulating heart rhythm. It has also been shown to reduce high blood pressure[12] which is one of the spokes on the insulin resistance wheel (see page 37).

Along with vitamin B6, zinc and biotin, magnesium is needed for the proper conversion of EFAs which produce anti-inflammatory prostaglandins (see page 72).

Best form to take

I'd suggest taking magnesium in supplement form as magnesium citrate as it is easier to absorb than the cheaper magnesium oxide.

Zinc

What does it do?

Zinc is needed for the production of stress hormones, insulin and sex hormones, and is crucial for maintaining healthy liver and immune function. Concentrated in the pancreas (where it helps to produce insulin), liver, bones, skin and kidneys, it is vital for our sense of taste and smell.

Zinc is also concentrated in muscles and it seems that the lower your zinc levels the less muscle mass you will have. Muscle is extremely important (see Chapter 6) as it helps to burn off fat, so a good zinc intake is crucial if you want to change your body shape.

If you are deficient in zinc, insulin cannot do its job properly and glucose cannot enter the cells. Because insulin levels then remain high in the blood, more insulin will be produced, leading to insulin resistance over time.

Zinc also affects a hormone called leptin which is produced by fat cells and controls appetite and hunger, telling us when we have had enough food. One study found that a zinc supplement increases the level of leptin[13] which can be helpful if you (like many) have a tendency to overeat.

Research has also shown that supplementing with zinc helps to control cortisol levels. In one study just 25–50mg of zinc prompted a significant fall in cortisol in healthy volunteers who had undergone an extreme exercise stress test that would normally raise cortisol.[14]

Another role of zinc is that together with vitamin B6, magnesium and biotin, it helps to convert the EFAs that produce the anti-inflammatory prostaglandins so helpful in offsetting the inflammatory effects of the fat around the middle.

Low zinc levels are associated with low sex drive which is one of the symptoms listed on page 18 in relation to stress hormones. So a supplement containing zinc could not only address the fat-around-the-middle problem, but also boost your libido.

Best form to take

Take zinc as zinc citrate or ascorbate rather than zinc oxide or sulphate as these are harder to absorb.

Manganese

What does it do?

Manganese is important for stimulating glycogen storage in the liver which helps to maintain a healthy blood sugar balance. It also has a role to play in metabolism and healthy thyroid function, and in helping the body to properly utilise vitamin C and the B vitamins.

Interestingly, if guinea pigs (which, like humans, do not manufacture their own vitamin C) become manganese deficient they develop diabetes. Diabetics tend to have only half the manganese levels of non-diabetics.

Best form to take

I would suggest taking manganese in the form of citrate or ascorbate for maximum absorption.

VITAL VITAMINS

Vitamin C

What does it do?

We know that vitamin C is involved with glucose metabolism and that, according to the Centre for Disease Control and Prevention in the USA, people with diabetes have significantly lower concentrations of vitamin C – up to 30 per cent lower in fact.[15] It is also thought that 'optimal vitamin C intake might help regulate blood sugar and aid in the prevention of diabetes'.[16]

Vitamin C can help to burn off that fat around the middle. Research has shown that people who have good levels of vitamin C burn 30 per cent more fat when doing moderate exercise than those who have low levels. It is thought that when vitamin C levels are low the body slows down the burning off of fat as a safety measure.[17]

Vitamin C is crucial for your adrenal gland function. The more cortisol you make, the more vitamin C you use and under stress you will excrete more vitamin C through urine. And don't forget, your body does not register what is triggering that stress – whether it is psychological (stuck in a traffic jam and fuming) or physical (blood sugar ups and downs) the effect on your body is the same and more vitamin C will be lost. So when you take vitamin C for a cold, it will also help your adrenal glands to respond to the stress of the infection.

Vitamin C is a water-soluble vitamin (as opposed to vitamin E for example which is fat soluble) and is transported into cells with the help of insulin. If insulin cannot do its job properly due to insulin resistance, you can end up with a vitamin C deficiency. Also, because vitamin C and glucose are very much alike in terms of their molecular structure it is thought that the two molecules end up competing with each other trying to get into the cells. So insulin resistance could prevent your body from using both glucose and vitamin C.

This is why it is thought that diabetics are frequently deficient in vitamin C. One study found that taking 2,000mg of vitamin C a day can lower glucose levels when combined with a healthy diet (see Chapter 4), avoiding sugar and refined carbohydrates.

Even a slight deficiency in vitamin C can trigger higher levels of cortisol[18] which in turn makes you more insulin resistant. A number of studies have shown that giving vitamin C to people undergoing stress (such as surgery or a sporting event) can bring cortisol levels back to normal fairly quickly. In one study, giving marathon runners vitamin C (1,000–1,500mg a day) for a week resulted in a 30 per cent lower cortisol level (compared to runners who were given a placebo).[19]

Vitamin C also helps to reduce cholesterol and lower blood pressure, two spokes on the insulin resistance wheel (see page 37).[20]

In the supplement programme (see page 163) I suggest using vitamin C together with flavonoids. These are found naturally in citrus fruits but they sit in the pith just under the fruit's skin. They are potent antioxidants and can control inflammation – crucial if your body is to let go of the fat around your middle because the extra weight registers as a low-grade inflammation.

Nearly all animals – except humans, apes and guinea pigs – manufacture their own vitamin C. We have to get it all from our diet and, sadly, we are not doing a good job; only 15 per cent of women are eating the recommended five a day fruit and vegetables.[21]

Best form to take

I suggest taking vitamin C in supplement form as an ascorbate, which is less acidic than the more common ascorbic acid. You will also need a higher dose than the RDA of 60mg. That was set as the level sufficient to prevent scurvy (a vitamin C deficiency disease) and is certainly not enough to help you to lose that fat around the middle or get you back into good health.

B vitamins

What do they do?

Water soluble like vitamin C, the B vitamins are known as the 'stress' vitamins. It is important to take them when you are working on nourishing and calming the adrenal function.

Vitamin B5 (pantothenic acid) is the most important B vitamin for your adrenal function. When you are under constant stress, your body's need for this vitamin will rise as it uses it to make the stress hormones, adrenaline and cortisol. Vitamin B5 helps in the conversion of glucose into energy. It is present in every cell in your body but in much higher concentrations in the adrenal glands because it is crucial in producing the adrenal hormones.

Vitamin B3 is also an important vitamin for the proper functioning of your adrenal glands and it helps to release energy from carbohydrates. It works with chromium to balance blood sugar. When you take chromium in the form of polynicotinate it is bound to vitamin B3 and is therefore helpful both for blood sugar and adrenals.

B vitamins also have an effect on blood sugar balance because they are needed for glucose metabolism. Biotin is one of the B vitamins needed for the synthesis of glucose. It has been shown to improve glucose control in those with Type 2 diabetes.[22] It is also needed for healthy nails and hair.

Vitamin B6 is needed for energy production and the metabolism of EFAs. Folic acid is another important B vitamin and, along with vitamins B6 and B12, it helps to control a substance called homocysteine. This is a toxic by-product from the breakdown of methionine (one of the essential amino acids) and it should, under normal circumstances, be detoxified (broken down and excreted) by the body. High levels of homocysteine have been linked to heart disease, Alzheimer's and osteoporosis, and research has also looked at whether there is a link between high homocysteine levels and high levels of insulin. In one study people with the metabolic syndrome (syndrome X, see page 30) were given both folic acid and B12. This combination not only reduced homocysteine levels as one would expect but also had a positive effect on insulin resistance.[23] It seems that the lower the level of homocysteine, the lower the level of insulin.

Best form to take

All the B vitamins (B1, B3, B6, B12 and folic acid) are needed for the release of energy from food so I recommend taking a supplement containing all the B vitamins. Your body needs other nutrients, such as magnesium, in order to convert B6 (as pyridoxine) into its active form (pyridoxal-5-phosphate), so try to take a supplement which offers B6 in the form of pyridoxal-5-phosphate just in case your body has trouble converting it from pyridoxine.

Vitamin E

What does it do?

Vitamin E is a fat-soluble antioxidant. It plays an important part in keeping your adrenal function healthy because when adrenal hormones are manufactured they create substances called free radicals.

During normal biochemical reaction, oxygen can become unstable, resulting in the 'oxidation' of other molecules. This, in turn, generates free radicals, and it is these that have been linked to premature ageing, cancer, coronary heart disease as well as to the brown patches on the skin of some elderly people. Free radicals speed up the ageing process by destroying healthy cells and they can also attack the DNA in the nucleus of a cell, causing cell mutation and cancer. They are also triggered by outside factors such as pollution, smoking, fried or barbecued food and UV rays from the sun.

Vitamin E mops up the free radicals that are produced inside the adrenal glands and elsewhere in the body, whilst vitamin C enhances the effects of the vitamin E.

Vitamin E also helps with glucose in a number of ways. Glucose itself increases free radical damage to cells and vitamin E can offset this with its antioxidant effect. It is crucial for people with insulin resistance because it improves the communication between insulin receptors and glucose as it makes the cell membranes more fluid.[24] When 600ius (international units) a day of vitamin E were given to diabetic patients it reduced both glucose levels and free-radical formation in only two weeks.[25] Vitamin E helps to control one of the inflammatory prostaglandins involved in platelet activation which causes blood to clot. That is one of the reasons why vitamin E has been shown to help reduce the risk of heart disease and stroke as it helps to prevent blood from clotting abnormally.

A study at Cambridge University showed that using 400–800ius of vitamin E a day helped to reduce the risk of a heart attack by 75 per cent. This was an eighteen-month trial involving 2,000 patients with coronary arteriosclerosis (fatty deposits in the arteries) of whom half were given a placebo.[26] It is thought that vitamin E prevents the 'bad' LDL from oxidising (or going off) in the blood.[27]

Best form to take

Vitamin E is a general term for tocopherols and there are four major kinds – alpha-, beta-, gamma- and delta-tocopherol. Alpha-tocopherol is the most common form, often found on its own in supplement form. However, for healthy adrenal function it is better to have a mix.

Generally speaking, I rate natural and synthetic vitamins equally because their molecular structures are identical. However, vitamin E as alpha-tocopherol is unusual in that the natural and synthetic forms are structurally different. The natural form is more biologically active, the body uses it much more easily and it is retained for longer in the body tissue, enabling it to perform its protective role. So when you buy vitamin E make sure that you have a very good look at the label. Choose one in which the alpha-tocopherol is in the natural form (d-alpha-tocopherol) and avoid the synthetic one (dl-alpha-tocopherol).

OTHER BENEFICIAL NUTRIENTS

There are some other extremely beneficial nutrients in this 'lose-your-belly' plan that may be taken in supplement form.

Essential fatty acids (EFAs)

What do they do?

I would say that most women, particularly those who follow no-fat and low-fat diets, do not get enough EFAs. They are, as their name implies, essential and your body cannot function healthily without them.

The Omega 3 essential fatty acids, EPA and DHA, have been shown to increase cell membrane responsiveness to insulin. One trial substituted just 7 per cent dietary fat with Omega 3 EFAs for four weeks. It reversed high levels of insulin being secreted in response to glucose[28] and this meant that 93 per cent of the fat content in the diet remained the same. This just shows how making small changes can make a huge difference.

In another study, a combination of fish oil (Omega 3) and chromium was given to obese rats. The combination of the two nutrients reversed the effects of both insulin resistance and also leptin resistance (in which the cells cannot use leptin, the hormone that controls appetite and hunger).[29]

Best form to take

I do not recommend taking either cod liver or halibut liver oil. The liver is the body's waste-disposal unit and fish can accumulate toxins and mercury which then have to pass through their livers. Oil that is extracted from the liver of the fish, therefore, is likely to contain higher quantities of these toxins than that taken from elsewhere in the body.

If you are vegetarian or simply prefer not to take fish oil, you can try taking linseed oil capsules. Linseed oil, also called 'flaxseed oil', contains the Omega 3 as well as some Omega 6 essential fatty acids. Your body has to convert linseed (flax) to EPA and DHA and this conversion can be blocked by the stress hormones, adrenaline and cortisol. It is also blocked by insulin, trans fats and too much saturated fat. In order for the conversion to take place, you also need good levels of zinc, magnesium, vitamin B6 and biotin (see the supplement programme on page 163). By reducing all the blocking factors and increasing the extra vitamin and minerals you will help your body convert the linseed (flax) oil into the nutrients it needs.

Co-enzyme Q10

What does it do?

This is a vitamin-like substance contained in nearly every cell of your body. It is important for energy production and normal carbohydrate metabolism. Deficiency in co-enzyme Q10 can occur with ageing and results in depleted energy levels.

Co-enzyme Q10 helps to shift fat around the middle because it releases energy by burning that fat. One study showed that people on a low-fat diet who took co-enzyme Q10 doubled their weight loss when compared with dieters not taking it.[30]

Co-enzyme Q10 also has a role to play in controlling blood sugar levels[31] and helps to lower glucose and insulin, so reversing insulin resistance. In one randomised double-blind trial patients with high blood pressure who were taking blood pressure medication were given co-enzyme Q10. On the Q10, they had lower levels of both glucose and insulin. But they also had lower blood pressure and triglycerides (blood fats). Their HDL ('good' cholesterol) also increased as did their levels of antioxidants, vitamins A, C, E and beta carotene. [32]

Co-enzyme Q10 also functions as an antioxidant and has other benefits, having been used to help heart problems and gum disease. In one study, 84 per cent of patients with heart failure showed significant improvements when 100mg per day of co-enzyme Q10 was included in their treatment.[33]

Alpha lipoic acid

What does it do?

Alpha lipoic acid is a powerful antioxidant that is made by the body and is a co-factor in vital energy-producing reactions. Its role is to release energy by burning glucose. It helps to make tissues more sensitive to insulin so that insulin can do its job of moving glucose into the cells and not storing it as fat.[34] Alpha lipoic acid also helps to support healthy liver function and because it is such a powerful antioxidant it has a role to play in slowing down the ageing process.

Research has also shown that alpha lipoic acid can prevent high blood pressure as well as preventing insulin resistance.[35]

> **WARNING**
>
> Consult your doctor before supplementing with alpha lipoic acid if you are diabetic and on medication. Because it can lower blood glucose levels, you will need to be monitored and your medication possibly altered accordingly.

Amino acids

What do they do?

Amino acids are the building blocks of the protein that you eat in your diet. There are twenty-five of them in all: eight are called 'essential' because they must be obtained from food, unlike the other seventeen which are made naturally by the body, by converting the essential ones.

Branched-chain amino acids (BCAAs) – what do they do?

This is a group of essential amino acids that include leucine, isoleucine and valine. They help with muscle growth and repair and also help to counteract the high levels of cortisol released when we are under stress. BCAAs can help to balance blood sugar and a deficiency of isoleucine can lead to symptoms identical to those of low blood sugar fluctuations e.g. irritability, mood swings and sugar cravings.

• FAT-BUSTING AMINO ACIDS •

Certain amino acids are vital to this programme because they can help to make cells more sensitive to insulin and others are important to help cushion the body against the effects of stress hormones.

Essential amino acids
Isoleucine*
Leucine*
Lysine
Methionine
Phenylalanine
Threonine
Trytophan
Valine*

Non-essential amino acids
Alanine
Arginine*
Aspartic acid
Carnitine*
Cysteine*
Cystine
GABA
Glutamic acid
Glutamine*
Glycine
Histidine
Homocysteine
Hydroxyproline
Proline
Serine
Taurine
Tyrosine*

* Fat-busting amino acids

Arginine – what does it do?

When it is under chronic stress your body cannot make enough of this amino acid for what it needs. Arginine is involved in promoting the release of blood sugar hormones including glucagon (the fat-burning hormone), so it is important to have good levels. It also helps with wound healing, the immune system, and heart health as it is involved with circulation and also liver function. The other valuable aspect of this amino acid is its role in muscle metabolism.

WARNING

Arginine should not be used if you are susceptible to herpes as it can trigger the virus.

Carnitine – what does it do?

Carnitine is involved in energy production and it helps by breaking down fat to release energy. As well as helping with losing that fat around the middle, carnitine is also essential for healthy heart function and deficiencies have been found in people with a number of heart conditions including angina and arrhythmia. This amino acid has also been shown to lower triglycerides (blood fats) and to increase HDL ('good') cholesterol and reduce LDL ('bad') cholesterol.

N-Acetyl cysteine – what does it do?

N-acetyl cysteine (NAC) is a form of the amino acid cysteine and is important in helping the metabolism of the Omega 3 fatty acids found in oily fish and linseed (flax). It is also a powerful antioxidant. Adding this to the diet as a supplement has been found to help reduce insulin levels and make the body more sensitive to insulin.[36] NAC has the added benefit of being helpful in eliminating heavy toxic metals like mercury, lead and cadmium from the body by binding to them and pulling them out.

WARNING

Consult your doctor before supplementing with n-acetyl cysteine if you are diabetic and on medication.

Glutamine – what does it do?

Like arginine, glutamine becomes essential when the body is under chronic stress. Normally the body can produce enough but stress creates such a need that the body cannot always provide it. The brain converts glutamine to glutamic acid which it needs to function properly. It can also help with sugar cravings as it can be converted to sugar for energy, so removing the need to eat something sweet. It was also shown, many years ago, to reduce the craving for alcohol.[37]

And to add to its benefits when shifting that weight around the middle, glutamine is the most abundant amino acid in the muscles of the body. It helps to build and maintain muscle which is critical when you want your body to burn fat. When you are under stress, the muscles release glutamine into the bloodstream and up to one third of the glutamine in the muscles can be released in this way. If you have enough glutamine when you are under stress, then you will not lose muscle mass and so weight (i.e. fat) loss becomes easier.

Tyrosine – what does it do?

Tyrosine is an amino acid synthesised by the body from phenylalanine. It is involved in suppressing appetite and helping to burn off fat. It plays an important part in the functioning of the adrenal and thyroid glands. Tyrosine has been studied by the US military for its effects on the body under stress. Personnel involved in combat training who were given tyrosine performed better in terms of concentration and memory than soldiers under the same stresses who were not given tyrosine.[38]

OTHER USEFUL SUPPLEMENTS

Green tea extract

What does it do?

Green tea (*Camellia sinensis*) contains many compounds including the polyphenols mentioned in the previous chapter. One of the categories of the polyphenols, catechins, have been shown to help burn off fat and also to inhibit growth of cancer cells by inducing cell death (apoptosis).[39]

Green tea also contains an amino acid called L-theanine which has a relaxing effect on the brain and body. Theanine causes an increase in alpha brain waves associated with being relaxed and alert but not wound up. Whereas beta waves can increase cortisol, alpha waves will reduce it.

Relaxation techniques and meditation can help your body to produce more alpha waves (see Chapter 7) and the theanine in green tea might also help.

Best form to take

I like to recommend a supplement (see page 163) containing a green tea extract instead of green tea itself during the initial three-month phase of your fat-loss programme, as you need to avoid the caffeine it contains.

Friendly, beneficial bacteria

What do they do?

When you eat refined carbohydrates, not only do they hit the bloodstream quickly causing a rise in blood sugar, more release of insulin and then the release of the stress hormones, they also change the environment in the gut enabling bacteria to survive and breed rather than passing through.

Unfriendly bacteria in the gut cause inflammation and the immune system responds by producing molecules called cytokines. Too many of these cytokines causes a problem because they can escape into the bloodstream and prevent insulin from binding on to the receptors, so contributing to insulin resistance.

We tend to think of the gut only in terms of our digestive system, but as much as 70 per cent of your immune system is located within the gut. So if you have a food intolerance your immune system will be doing battle with foods it sees as foreign and producing cytokines to fight them. Yeasts will also cause an immune response as will parasites (see page 183 for information on how to test for these).

All food must be broken down by the digestive system, passed into the bloodstream and dealt with by the body. If this does not happen properly, the body 'sees' normal food as an antigen, a toxin, and sets up an immune system reaction to deal with it. At the same time, the undigested food is sitting around fermenting and putrefying. Large spaces can develop between the cells in the gut wall and food molecules can then pass into the bloodstream. This is called leaky gut or 'intestinal permeability'.

Stress has a direct effect on the gut and can make the body react to ordinary foods that you have eaten for years without any problems. And because stress affects the immune system it allows unfriendly bacteria and yeast to thrive.

So you need to do two things: add in good amounts of beneficial bacteria and take out any foods that might be causing your body to react. Refined foods such as white bread, cakes and biscuits should be the first to go. Also, if you think you may be reacting to something like wheat or milk, then it is worth doing a test to find out (see page 183).

Best form to take

Despite the huge amount of money pumped into advertising 'friendly bacteria' drinks I feel it's better to take yours in supplement form as the levels are far more concentrated and help to re-colonise the gut more quickly. The drinks are often loaded with sugar which just adds to the problem you're trying to solve, first, by causing a rise in blood sugar and second by feeding negative bacteria and yeast in the gut.

HEALTHY HERBS

Do herbs really help?

In 2003, an analysis of 108 clinical trials using thirty-six herbs and nine vitamin/mineral supplements on over 4,000 patients with diabetes or poor glucose control showed an improvement in the control of blood sugar in more than 75 per cent of cases.[40] So which herbs are useful for getting rid of fat around the middle?

Siberian ginseng (Eleutherococcus senticosus)

What does it do?

There are a number of herbs with a long history of helping with adrenal function and calming the body. So whilst you are being diligent about your diet and getting your blood sugar under control, herbs can soothe the adrenal glands. The herb of choice for the adrenal glands is Siberian ginseng. It is classed as an adaptogen, which means that it works according to your body's need – providing energy when required, and helping to combat stress and fatigue when you are under pressure. It helps to encourage the normal functioning of the adrenals and acts as a tonic to these glands.[41]

Siberian ginseng is different from Panax ginseng (also called Asian, Chinese or Korean ginseng). Panax ginseng is more potent than Siberian ginseng and is often more suitable for men as it has a much stronger effect on boosting energy. In some women it is strong enough to cause palpitations and should only be used in the short term (just a few weeks). Siberian ginseng on the other hand is a very nourishing herb for the adrenal glands and can be used over three to six months if you have been under constant stress.

Rhodiola (Rhodiola rosea)

What does it do?

Like Siberian ginseng, rhodiola is classed as an adaptogen, so it has a balancing effect on the body and at the same time helps to combat stress caused by the pressures of modern-day life. It has been shown to help boost energy, improve memory and may also act like a herbal antidepressant.

In one study, rhodiola was tested against a placebo in students during stressful exams. Their physical and mental performance was assessed before and after the exams.[42] Students taking the rhodiola coped better generally with the stress of the exams and experienced less mental fatigue.

Rhodiola has also been given to hospital doctors working night shifts to see the effect it had on their ability to perform certain tasks and their level of fatigue. The doctors took the herb for two weeks and it was found that their mental performance improved in areas such as short-term memory, calculations, ability to concentrate even when under stress from sleep deprivation and their energy levels also were better than they were without the herb.[43]

Best form to take

There are different species of rhodiola herb and it is important to make sure that you use *Rhodiola rosea* as this is the kind that has the stress-busting properties.

Valerian (Valeriana officinalis)

What does it do?

Sleep is important for losing that fat around the middle because there is a link between not getting enough sleep and higher cortisol levels (see Chapter 7 on stress). If stress is affecting your sleep the herb valerian can be very helpful. It is classed as a sedative in herbal medicine and not only helps with insomnia but can also promote relaxation and reduce anxiety and tension. It is best taken just before bed.

> **WARNING**
>
> Do not use valerian if you are taking sleeping pills.

HERBS TO AVOID

There are some herbs that should be avoided when you are aiming to lose weight around the middle:

Liquorice (Glycyrrhiza glabra)

Although this herb is known as an anti-stress herb and would, in most circumstances, be recommended, one of the compounds in liquorice (glycyrrhizin) is metabolised in the body to molecules whose structure is similar to that of the adrenal hormones. It has the ability to prevent the breakdown of cortisol so keeping the levels high. People with adrenal exhaustion and low cortisol may find that liquorice increases energy, but when you are trying to trim an apple shape, you need to lower cortisol levels, so it's better to avoid liquorice.

Deglycyrrhizinated licorice (DGL) has had the glycyrrhizin removed. It is used mainly to help with digestive problems as it soothes the oesophagus (food pipe) and stomach.

Stimulant herbs

A number of herbs found in 'weight loss' products have a stimulant effect on the body, in effect speeding it up and also stimulating the central nervous system which can increase heart rate, blood pressure and nervousness. These amphetamine-like stimulants include:

- ma haung (*Ephedra sinensis*)
- guarana (*Paullinia cupana*)
- yohimbine (*Pausinystalia yohimbe*)

They work in exactly the same way as caffeine, by giving you a boost so that you feel you have more energy. They also increase adrenaline and cortisol which is why you should avoid them.

There is no quick fix to losing weight, especially the weight around your middle, because your body has been told that it needs to keep hold of it to protect your life from danger. Weight-loss products – herbal or otherwise – will never work in the long term.

The list of vitamins, minerals and other nutrients you need may seem long but you can get many of them in one good multivitamin and mineral, and just take the others as extras. See Chapter 10, 'Plan of Action', for a complete, easy-to-use supplement plan.

• Chapter 6 •

EXERCISE THAT'S BEST FOR YOU

Why apple shapes need to build up muscle as well as a good sweat

We all know that exercise is good for us. It keeps our heart healthy, helps to keep the bowels working efficiently, improves the function of the immune system and releases endorphins (the 'feel-good' chemicals) in the brain. But all too many of us are just not doing enough of it. The British Heart Foundation estimates that a third of all adults do not even take thirty minutes of vigorous exercise a week, let alone the thirty minutes a day they recommend.

Why is this? Well, just a generation ago exercise was a part of everyday life. You didn't have to make a conscious effort to go to the gym. People walked a few miles each day either to work or school. Household chores that we now organise with the flick of a switch required considerably more effort. Shopping was done almost daily and in different shops, without the convenience of supermarkets where you could buy a whole week's supplies in one go, let alone Internet shopping (which exercises the fingers only).

Life in general was physically more demanding, and our parents and grandparents really had no choice but to be active. At the same time it was mentally and emotionally less demanding. Life was taken at a slower pace because tasks took longer to complete. You couldn't pop a meal into the microwave and have it on the table in ten minutes, television was for many people a luxury and shops were closed in the evenings and on Sundays.

There is no doubt that life in the twenty-first century is filled with conveniences. But it really is so unhealthy. Everything we do is so fast-paced, frantic and stressful, yet many of us do nothing more energetic than walking up stairs to bed. The sedentary nature of modern life means that our body's stress response is more acute than ever before.

As I have explained in earlier chapters, when the stress hormones cortisol and adrenaline are released into your bloodstream, your body expects you to run or fight for your life. But the stress of being stuck on a train when you are late for an appointment cannot be mitigated by any form of physical activity. You just have to sit there and stew and there is no physical release for the hormones. With no option for activity, they urge the body to eat or drink.

Exercise or physical activity has never been more important. If you have fat around the middle of your body caused, in part, by your stress hormones, exercise has to be a priority. It's not hard, but it is vital, and following the specific exercise recommendations in this chapter you will benefit by:

- burning off fat around the middle
- reducing the negative effects of both cortisol and insulin
- increasing your muscle mass (which in turn burns calories)
- burning calories and using body fat (everywhere in the body) as fuel
- preventing and even reversing insulin resistance
- reducing blood sugar and insulin
- improving insulin sensitivity in skeletal muscles and fat
- improving your body shape

Don't allow yourself to get too hung up on your weight – remember that you want to lose fat, not just weight. With the focus on fat around your middle you should not expect dramatically rapid results as you cannot lose more than a pound or two of fat a week. The changes will be subtle at first but after just a couple of weeks on my plan you will start to notice a change in body shape.

The first change that women who have followed my plan notice is that they start to feel much flatter under the bust. After this, clothes start to feel looser around the waist. These are all signs that the plan is working. Ignore the scales as this can – and often does – happen without you actually losing weight. This is because when you exercise properly you will gain muscle, and muscle weighs more than fat. However, a pound of fat takes up about five times as much space as a pound of muscle so as your fat levels go down and your muscle mass goes up you will start to look smaller. You could even drop a dress size whilst still staying the same weight.

When assessing your progress, remember that measuring and keeping track of your body fat percentage is a much more accurate measurement than BMI (see page 25).

THE IMPORTANCE OF MUSCLE

If you cut right back on calories or go on a severely restrictive diet, your body will go into survival mode. This becomes a stress in itself and your body will do all it can to hold on to body fat for protection. You may lose weight rapidly by eating nothing but lettuce and pineapple, but the weight you lose will be made up of at least 25–30 per cent muscle and water, not just fat.

Muscle plays a really important role in helping to control your weight and you can't afford to lose it. In fact, not only do you not want to lose it, you really need to try to put a bit more on. And the good news is that muscle is metabolically active. This means it requires fuel in the form of calories just to maintain it even when you sit and do nothing. So the more muscle you have, the more calories you consume, and, if you do not overeat, the more fat you will burn:

450g (1lb) of muscle burn 75 calories a day
450g (1lb) of fat burn 8 calories a day

This is one of the reasons why men, infuriatingly, find it easier to lose weight than women. It's all to do with their build. They generally have more muscle than women and can, therefore, burn calories faster – even when they are doing nothing. Furthermore, higher levels of male sex hormones, like testosterone, mean that they can build muscle faster through exercise.

When your body is under stress and cortisol levels go up, it uses muscle for fuel to provide energy. Cortisol breaks down muscle turning it into amino acids, the building blocks of the protein that you eat. Your liver then turns these amino acids into fuel – the higher your cortisol level (and the longer it remains high, under ongoing stress), the more muscle will be broken down to supply glucose for fuel. And, as we have seen, the higher the glucose level, the more insulin is produced to combat it. Over time this increases the risk of insulin resistance with all its associated health problems (see page 36).

To compound this, the fact that muscle is being broken down means that there is less muscle to burn fat. So your metabolism slows down and, although you are trying to lose weight, you will get progressively fatter.

WHY EXERCISE ALONE IS NOT ENOUGH

It would be lovely to think that all your fat-around-the-middle problems could be solved by merely upping the exercise rather than having to make changes in your life as a whole, by controlling stress and altering the way in which you eat. Exercise does make a big difference to your overall health and will make the whole process quicker and more efficient, but it's just not going to do it on its own.

• WEIGHT GAIN WITH AGE •

It is sad but true that we all tend to gain weight as we get older. One of the main reasons is that we lose muscle. After the age of forty, women can start to lose about 225g (8oz) of muscle a year. Inactive women over the age of forty lose muscle mass twice as fast as inactive men. So over ten years between the ages of forty and fifty, most of us will have lost 2.25kg (5lb) in muscle. With decreasing muscle mass our metabolism becomes increasingly sluggish and, let's face it, we all also tend to get less active as we get older in any case. This inactivity will only add to the problem and with less muscle and less activity weight is likely to pile on as fat.

Exercise alone may be enough for some men. But women are built differently with less muscle and extra fat so it is harder to shift that fat. One study followed the progress of seventy-four overweight men and women aged between seventeen and thirty-five over a sixteen-month period. They asked half the group to follow an exercise regime and the other half to continue with their normal activity levels. Neither group was asked to change their diet. At the end of the study, the men following the exercise regime lost an average of almost 5kg (11lb). Some of the women lost weight but others gained weight and on average the women ended up weighing the same. But the women in the group that did not follow the exercise regime ended up gaining an average of around 3.25kg (7lb) in weight over that time.[1] The results of this study prove just why you need to put into place not only the exercise recommendations but also the lifestyle, diet and supplement advice in this book to make a real difference.

WHAT KIND OF EXERCISE IS BEST?

Aerobic or anaerobic?

In order to lose that fat around the middle, you need to do a combination of two types of exercise, cardiovascular (getting you puffed) and resistance-training (with weights or bands to build muscles).[2] The aim is to use exercise to help burn off fat and to build muscle which helps you to burn off even more fat and faster.

Aerobic exercise (also known as cardiovascular exercise) means 'with oxygen'. Anaerobic exercise, also known as weight-training or resistance-training, means 'without oxygen'. It is any exercise that puts your muscles under tension e.g. using weight machines at the gym, dumbbells at home or exercises like press-ups or lunges.

There has been much debate in the exercise world as to whether aerobic or anaerobic exercise is the best way to help you to lose body fat. It has been said that you can burn more calories in thirty minutes of aerobic exercise than you can in thirty minutes of weight-training. This is true but we have to look at the bigger picture.

I recommend an exercise programme that not only burns off the calories whilst you are exercising but one that changes the message to your body to stop storing fat and start burning it off as energy. The fastest and most effective way to do this is to combine aerobic and anaerobic exercise.

Weight-training will help you to lose more body fat over a twenty-four-hour period than aerobic activity alone. This is because aerobic exercise only helps to burn fat for about eight hours after the exercise, whereas anaerobic exercise builds muscle which continues to burn fat even whilst you are asleep.

By doing weight-training you build muscle which revs up your metabolism and increases your basal metabolic rate (BMR). This is the amount of calories

• ARE AEROBICS REALLY THE ANSWER? •

Aerobic exercise is crucial for making your cells more receptive to insulin. And you don't have to drop everything to train for a marathon. Even modest exercise can make a significant difference.[3] Aerobic exercise also significantly lowers homocysteine levels so by making it a part of your life you will automatically reduce your risk of heart disease, stroke, osteoporosis and Alzheimer's.[4]

However, frustratingly, although research into many of the weight-loss studies has shown that the supposed holy grail of combining diet and aerobic exercise *does* lead to weight loss, it gives you only a slight advantage over women who diet without exercising at all.[5]

It can be really demoralising and depressing to exercise religiously twice or three times a week (as so many people do) and not see any improvement. And that's why so many people give up.

The only way to get results is to do the *right* kind of exercise and the right combination.

Thirty minutes of pounding a treadmill three times a week (a typical recommendation) only uses up about 187 calories. One pound of body fat contains the equivalent of 3,555 calories, so if you made no dietary changes[6] you'd have to do nineteen sessions just to lose one pound of fat!

Even if you combine aerobics with the dietary recommendations in Chapter 4, you may still not be on the right track; you could end up *losing* muscle because your body will be tempted to break down muscle to fuel your aerobic exercise instead of using your plentiful fat reserves. If aerobic exercise is done for a short period of time, less than twenty minutes, then the body uses carbohydrate for fuel and not fat and it gets that by breaking down muscle.

But don't be disheartened. The good news is that once you have changed your body shape and that fat around the middle has gone, good old aerobic exercise is great for keeping your new shape.[7]

you burn every day simply by being alive. So the more you increase your BMR the more chance you have of losing fat even whilst you are doing nothing. Muscle requires energy so the more muscle you have, the more fuel you burn. Fat does not require any energy to maintain it.

Don't worry, you won't end up looking like Arnie and you are not going to be using huge weights. The aim is that as you use the weights or do resistance exercises your body uses your stored fat to build muscles and increase your metabolism. The tension caused by the exercises causes slight damage to the muscles which then repair themselves after the workout, which is when they grow. This growth requires a significant amount of energy so when the repair takes place whilst you are sleeping, you will actually be losing body fat to supply the energy needed for the repair.

Let's look at the evidence comparing aerobic exercise to weight-training for burning off fat. In one study, thirty minutes of exercise a day over an eight-week period was split between one group who did half aerobic exercise and half weight-training and another group who just did aerobic. The participants following the combined exercise programme lost 3.25kg (7lb) more fat than the group doing just aerobics.[8]

And what about weight-training combined with dietary changes? A study at Tufts University in America gave women a similar diet to the one I'm recommending (to encourage slow but steady weight loss) and half of the women also followed a weight-training programme twice a week. Both sets of women lost around 5.8kg (13lb) in weight. However, when their body fat measurements were taken, the difference between the two groups of women was striking. The women in the diet-only group lost around 1.3kg (3lb) of muscle along with the fat but those who had also done the weight-training programme gained around 450g (1lb) of muscle. So all the weight they lost was actually fat – a total of 44 per cent more than the diet-only group[9] – and they completely changed their body shape.

Your body is very clever. In the same way that it adapts to any restriction in food by slowing the metabolism it also adapts to exercise. So after about four weeks of doing one sort of exercise it becomes more efficient and uses less energy to perform the same activity. To maintain the same fat-burning impact you have to continually change the exercise you are doing (walking to running, then cycling, then rowing etc.), increasing the intensity to trick your body out of its normal patterns.

The best way to prevent your body from adapting to aerobic exercise is to vary the intensity of the activity with interval training (see Chapter 10).

Yoga, t'ai chi and qi gong

All these forms of activity can be really helpful as part of your fat-loss programme because they also act as stress-busters and lower cortisol levels in the body. They all involve slow, controlled movements with a focus on breathing correctly, which can be very calming. Without realising it, many people have a tendency to shallow-breathe, which is effectively what happens in the fight-or-flight response, and in times of stress it can lead to hyperventilating. Yoga and other similar exercise classes can help to teach you the correct way to breathe. Yoga is also a form of resistance-training in which your own body weight provides the resistance.

Pilates

Although the Pilates body-conditioning system has been around for about eighty years it has gained widespread popularity in the last decade. It was originally devised after the First World War by Joseph Pilates, a German nurse and physical therapist to help bedridden patients to recover their muscle strength.

Pilates exercises are performed on the floor or on specialised equipment and their aim is to teach body self-awareness, to strengthen muscles (especially in the back and abdomen) without straining them and to improve flexibility. It is best described as a combination of yoga and weight-training.

Pilates and exercises performed on large stability balls can help to improve what is called core stability – they are helpful in strengthening the muscles around the middle (core strength). Core muscles lie deep within the upper body torso and the stability exercises focus on working all these deep muscles at the same time. The exercises must be taught properly so it is worthwhile joining a class, having individual instruction or getting a good video.

Alexander technique and Feldenkrais method

Both of these are 'body awareness' methods that teach you how to use your core strength. Tension in the body can be created from actions as simple as sitting, standing, turning and breathing. These techniques re-educate the body to move as efficiently and effortlessly as it was designed to do. Both methods involve unlearning bad postural habits and improving the way in

Quick-fix Stomach Trimmers

If you have spent many years with excess fat around your middle, the chances are that you would have been tempted at one time or another by the many stomach-trimming gadgets on the market. Wouldn't it be wonderful if you could ignore all my advice and, instead, just wrap a piece of rubber around your tummy, switch it on and achieve the same effect? Sadly these devices just cannot have the same impact.

Stomach crunches (or sit-ups) cannot do the job alone either. Of course, it is important to keep your abdominals strong with core stability exercises and crunches, but don't expect localised exercise to solve the problem. When your stomach muscles are completely covered in a thick layer of fat, any six-pack you may be working on simply won't show until the fat has gone.

The only way to lose fat is by giving your body a new message. The problem can only be solved from the inside out.

which you hold yourself. You can actually look slimmer just by standing properly and not slouching!

IT'S BAD NOT TO EXERCISE

The benefits of exercise are enormous. You will gain the body shape you want and lose that fat around your middle because the exercise is helping you in a number of ways. After as few as ten minutes of strenuous exercise the brain produces endorphins (the feel-good neurotransmitters) that calm you down and decrease stress hormone levels. Research has shown that just brisk walking four times a week reduces body fat, lowers insulin resistance and reduces food consumption.[10]

If you are exercising now for the first time, or for the first time in years, it would be best to join a local gym so that professionals can show you how to exercise and what level to start at.

The benefits of exercise hold true across all age groups and both sexes so there is never a good enough reason *not* to start, especially when it is so clear that the combination of diet and exercise is even more effective for weight loss than either intervention alone.[11] (See Chapter 10, 'Plan of Action', for a complete easy-to-use exercise plan.)

• Chapter 7 •

Just How Stressed Are You?

'The mind is its own place and in itself can
make a hell of heaven, a heaven of hell.'
Paradise Lost, John Milton

As is quite clear by now, the real key to getting rid of the weight around your middle is by reducing levels of the stress hormones, especially cortisol, and as I have explained over the course of the past few chapters, you can achieve this by making a number of changes in your life at the same time. These include:

- keeping your blood sugar in balance by following my dietary recommendations
- taking a programme of supplements for three months
- taking time to exercise

However, in order for all the above changes to be effective, it is crucial that you also take a good look at the stress in your life to ascertain what you can and cannot control.

Although we live in a high-tech, high-convenience world in which we have access to twenty-four-hour shopping and television and a machine to perform just about every possible daily task, we are all increasingly time-poor, not time-rich as you might expect. With everyone using mobile phones, texting and e-mailing, there is a constant call for immediate responses and results, creating ongoing demands and pressure.

For many women the feeling is that there is, quite simply '**No time for me**'.

It is estimated that three quarters of British women aged between twenty-five and fifty-five suffer from the stress-related Hurried Woman Syndrome caused by taking care of everybody but themselves. It is a modern-day phenomenon with the classic symptoms of tiredness, increased appetite and a lack of sex drive – all of which are also associated with excess cortisol.

You might find that you, like so many women, perform the equivalent of a constant juggling act with countless plates spinning in the air. Each plate represents one of several different demands: work, partner, children, housework, caring for elderly relatives. You spend your life desperately keeping those plates spinning because if you do not, they will all come crashing down.

It may not all be earth-shattering, deadline-looming, multi-million-pound business stress, but it is very, very tough. And it's relentless.

Your body does not differentiate between the stress of getting three young children out of the house each morning, rescuing a multi-million pound company from near ruin, or running for your life. A stress is a stress is a stress. The physical effects are the same, whatever the cause, and it is extremely bad for your health.

If you have a tendency to gather fat around your middle, there is a very strong chance you are under stress. Your body is simply trying to cushion you against the onslaught that is your everyday life.

You may see no end to it, but this way of life cannot go on indefinitely. Something will have to give, otherwise you will find yourself slipping slowly down the ill-health slope towards heart disease, high blood pressure or diabetes (see page 36). For the sake of your health – if not your figure – you need to take stock of your life, and consider what changes need to be made.

It need not be as hard as you might think. Simply by getting your blood sugar levels under control (using my 'lose-your-belly' eating plan) you will automatically reduce part of the stress load on your body as you will be stepping off that rollercoaster of blood sugar highs and crashing lows (see page 51). It's a great first step and once you have done it you will feel as if you have more control over your life and you will be able to make the sort of changes that will reduce the stress response further still. So often women tell me that sorting out their diet made them feel much more able to cope.

LOOK AT YOUR LIFE

There are two ways of tackling the stress in your life. Either bite the bullet and make a few really big changes so that you no longer have to juggle so much (cut your working hours, go to bed earlier and get up earlier in the morning so that you are not so rushed) or learn a few coping strategies to help you change the way you handle stress, and lessen its physical impact.

Take a few minutes to have a careful look at your life and consider the following questions:

- Are there any stressful factors you could fundamentally change?
- If your job is simply too stressful perhaps should you consider changing it?
- Do you have unrealistic expectations or goals?
- Are you putting yourself under too much pressure to be some kind of Superwoman?
- Do you really have to do everything?
- What can you change externally?
- Is there anything you can do to change your attitude to life?
- Can you learn to say 'No'?

A really great step in the right direction would be learning to manage your time more effectively. You could do this by:

- sitting down to plan out a weekly schedule
- making a weekly meal plan so that you are not caught on the hop with hungry children
- allowing yourself a little more time with family or friends (one night a week with the girls perhaps?)
- allocating a little time each week, or each day, to relax doing something you enjoy doing (even if it's just one Sudoku, it's *your* treat)

Taking control of your time in this way is not an indulgence – it is important to do it and worth the effort involved in making it happen. It will help you to avoid falling into yet another stress trap, running late, missing appointments, eating on the run and never quite making time for yourself.

Parkinson's Law states that 'work expands to fill the time available'. Try to put this into practice. Take a little time for yourself and see what happens: your world will not collapse – everything else will just have to fit in around you. The fact is, the less stressed you are, the more you will actually achieve in a shorter space of time because your body and mind will be functioning at peak efficiency and not in some sort of blind panic, where you cannot think straight.

Make a few changes right now. Maybe you could think about downshifting, perhaps? Could you change jobs or put in a pitch for working at home one day a week? How about paying for a little stress relief and getting some extra help with the house or the children? By putting the emphasis on your own health and well-being, you could put yourself back in control of your life.

Think of yourself as the heart of your family, pumping away keeping everyone happy and healthy. But the human heart is selfish and in times of trouble it will always ensure that it is nourished with blood and oxygen before any other organ – if it wasn't, the other organs would not survive. Similarly, you owe it to your nearest and dearest to look after yourself, because without you they would never manage. Give yourself permission to think about you.

You may remember that I quoted Hans Selye earlier in the book saying, 'No one can live without experiencing some degree of stress all the time…' (see page 16). There is a rule called the Yerkes–Dodson Law which states that health and performance increase proportionately, as a result of stress, up to a point called the 'optimum stress point', beyond which they crash back down.

The law explains why it is just as bad to have too little stress as it is to have too much. As with everything in the body, a balance is required. With too little stress, we would not get out of bed in the morning; we need some stress just to motivate us.

At the optimum stress point (the top of the curve) you really are in 'the zone', where the stress level is just right – remember those days when you

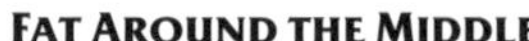

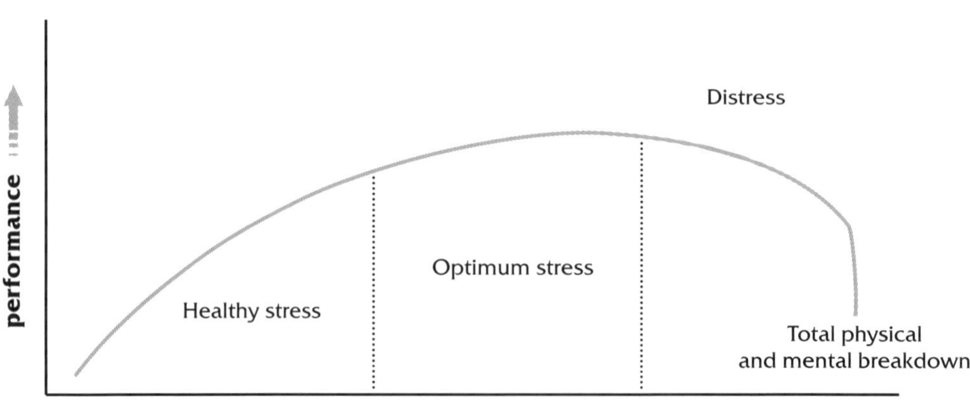

could get up and just get everything done with seemingly minimal effort? As stress tips over that point, you might not even notice the change at first, except that it may take you a little longer to get things done. But then a simple thing can go wrong (not finding a parking space which might just make you late) and suddenly everything seems to fall apart. That's when you realise that you are not coping and that you cannot carry on like this.

Except that most people do struggle on. And increasing waistlines across the nation are testimony to that.

Have a look at the diagram above. Where are you on the curve? If you've gone beyond your 'comfort zone' just stop and think: what can you do to get your stress levels back where they should be?

STRESS-BUSTING TIPS

Prioritise

Make a long, long list of all your stressful tasks and prioritise them in order of importance. All too often the most difficult or onerous tasks get put off, but just think how much better you would feel, and how much freer your mind would be if those tough tasks were done. As you do each task tick it off.

Delegate

Try to let other people do things for you when you can. It is a very female characteristic to try to do everything yourself because nobody can do it quite as well. If this 'lose-your-belly' plan is going to work, you need to let go so that your body will let go of that fat as well.

Put yourself first

It is important to do this at least some of the time. You could decide that exercise is *your* time and make a point of allowing space to do it. Better still, book yourself a regular massage. This will be time for *you*, giving it double stress-busting impact as massage will help to lower your cortisol levels.[1] Other natural therapies can also reduce the stress hormones. For example, the World Health Organisation recognises acupuncture as an appropriate treatment for stress, whilst reflexology, yoga and t'ai chi are all widely used to help the relaxation process. Find a therapy that works for you – try them all. You may find that the process of experimenting with various treatments is relaxing in itself!

Start small – even as little as ten minutes for yourself a day – and build up. Read a magazine, do a crossword puzzle, and build up until you spend a proportion of every day doing what *you* want to do.

Learn some relaxation techniques

This can be as simple as just listening to some soothing music, indulging in a hot bath with aromatherapy oils, taking a peaceful walk or practising yoga or meditation. Meditation has been shown to be effective for both reducing stress and lowering high blood pressure.[2] You could also try learning a visualisation technique or learning to breathe slowly.

PROGRESSIVE MUSCLE RELAXATION

This is a wonderful relaxation technique that costs nothing and that you can do on your own at home. But you must allow the time to do it. Find a quiet space, shut the door, unplug the phone and take a few deep breaths:

Lying on your back, tense each part of your body as you breathe in. Then hold your breath for five seconds, keeping your muscles tense. Relax and breathe out again slowly over a count of about ten seconds.

Curl your toes up and press down with your feet. Relax.

Press your heels down, pulling your toes up. Relax.

Tense your calf muscles. Relax.

Straighten your legs and tense your thigh muscles. Relax.

Tighten your buttocks. Relax.

Tighten your stomach muscles. Relax.

Bend your elbows up and flex your biceps. Relax.

Hunch your shoulders and tense your neck muscles. Relax.

Clench your teeth, frown and screw up your eyes as tight as you can. Relax.

Tense all the muscles at the same time. After ten seconds, relax.

Now close your eyes. Concentrate your mind for thirty seconds on an imaginary diamond glinting on a black velvet background, whilst continuing to breathe slowly and deeply.

Now focus on another peaceful object of your choice for thirty seconds.

Open your eyes.

• PUT THINGS IN PERSPECTIVE •

Are the things you worry about *really* that important in the wider scheme of things? As Mark Twain said, 'I am an old man and have known many troubles, but most never happened.' It has been said that 40 per cent of our worries never happen and 40 per cent of what happens we can do nothing about; that adds up to 80 per cent of 'stuff' that there is just no point in worrying about!

Take time to eat

Don't eat on the run or put off eating in order to get something else done. The process of *how* you eat is as important as *what* you eat (see page 76). I know many women who get up and down from the table during a meal because they are serving and fetching things for other family members. Stop! Take your time, sit down and take a few deep breaths before you start eating, then chew your food well and do not drink whilst you are eating. Savour your food, taking time to enjoy the taste and smells. By taking a little longer to eat you will end up eating less food automatically because you will be allowing your body the twenty minutes needed for your brain to register that you are full.

You must also try to stop using food as a way of coping with stress. When you are under stress your body will tell you to eat, and although it is a very strong impulse, you need to break that cycle.

Take time to go to the toilet

As obvious as this might sound, it is often quite easy to be too busy to sit and poo properly because you are rushing around doing other things! Your body needs a routine and so do your bowels. You need to pass a bowel motion at least once a day as this is your body's way of getting rid of toxins and waste products. A gastroenterologist once remarked that men are more likely to pass a more complete bowel motion than women, as they often sit there for a while reading the paper and don't get up until they have finished.

Take regular exercise

This is important for the body in terms of shifting that weight around the middle (see Chapter 6), but it is equally as important for the mind. Exercise helps to release neurotransmitters called endorphins, which make us feel happier, more alert and calm. It also helps to suppress the appetite for a while afterwards because you have used up stress hormones and your body is no longer telling you to eat. Studies show that exercise can reduce the impact of stress, raise self-esteem, relieve anxiety and depression and improve mood.[3]

Exercise – in stress-busting terms – does not have to be a five-mile run; it can be as simple as dancing at home to music you enjoy and singing at the same time if you can manage it!

Have a cuddle

Mums have always known that a cuddle works wonders and now scientists have confirmed that hugging can reduce stress because it helps to raise oxytocin levels. A study looked at the levels of oxytocin and adrenaline before and after couples had a cuddle. A twenty-second cuddle lowered adrenaline and increased levels of oxytocin.[4]

Keep laughing

Make sure you keep your sense of humour. It has been shown that if you can smile and laugh even when you may not feel like it, your body releases feel-good chemicals that can bring about a positive change in mood. Laughter increases the supply of oxygen in the blood, which can influence the feel-good neurotransmitters in the brain, making you feel happier. So laughter really is the best medicine!

Learn to breathe

This is one of the most important stress-busting tips of them all. You might wonder why you need to learn to breathe – surely we do that automatically? But breathing correctly is a different matter. If you watch a baby breathe, you will see that their whole abdomen rises and falls as they breathe, because they are breathing with their diaphragm. But we, as adults, tend to shallow-breathe using just the top half of the chest which makes us more tense and also tired.

When you are stressed you are more likely to shallow-breathe which can actually increase feelings of stress. It is almost like hyperventilating. By learning to breathe with your diaphragm (belly-breathing), you will not only be signalling to your body that you are less stressed, but you will also be circulating more oxygen around your body and mind. This will give you more energy, allow the feel-good neurotransmitters in the brain to do their job efficiently and also activate the relaxation centres in the brain.

• DO YOU SHALLOW-BREATHE OR BELLY-BREATHE? •

Lie down on your back. Put your right hand on your chest and your left hand over your belly button. Breathe as you would normally. Watch your hands and see which one moves more with each breath. If the right hand is moving more than the left you are a shallow- (or chest-) breather and this needs to change.

By breathing correctly you can reduce levels of cortisol, allowing your body to let go of the weight around the middle. But that's not all. You burn your food in the presence of oxygen, so with more oxygen circulating in your body you will be able to burn your food even more efficiently. This automatically gives you more energy, increases the metabolism and stops the body from storing food as fat.

Some exercises – yoga and Pilates, for example – teach you how to breathe correctly but you can also learn to do this at home. As with anything new, it will feel slightly strange at first but it should become as automatic as the shallow-breathing you have been doing until now.

Start with this simple exercise for ten minutes each day over the next week:

1. Lie on your stomach with your legs approximately 60cm (2ft) apart and your feet relaxed outwards.
2. Fold your arms, place your hands on your biceps and your head on your arms.
3. Relax.

Because of the pressure from the floor, you will only be able to breathe through your diaphragm, so just feel your breathing for the next ten minutes:

- Your breath should flow smoothly in and out.
- The out-breath should be longer than the in-breath.
- You should be breathing through your nose and not your mouth.

Once you have the done this ten minutes daily for a week, try it standing upright:

1. Stand with your feet slightly apart.
2. Take a few gentle breaths in and out through your nose.
3. Place your hands over your belly.
4. As you breathe in, push your belly out – you should be able to feel your hands being pushed out.
5. Pause briefly.
6. Breathe out slowly through your nose.
7. As you breathe out, imagine all the tension and stress leaving your body just like a soft flowing stream.
8. Repeat ten times.

Try to do this every day over the next three months.

Get enough sleep

Sleep plays an extremely important part in a healthy lifestyle, and far too many of us get too little. Stress and sleep are inversely related – the less sleep you get, the more difficulty you will find in adapting to challenging situations; the more sleep you have, the less stressful everyday pressures seem.

Sleep is not only important for your overall health, but it is also essential for ensuring that your body is working at its best and that you are physically and emotionally able to cope with the demands of day-to-day living. Sleep gives your body time to recharge its batteries, enabling tissue repair and cell growth to take place. A lack of sleep is perceived as yet another stress by the body.

As a society, we have pushed the waking day to its limit and sleep has become almost a luxury, rather than the necessity it really is. The amount of sleep we get is constantly decreasing. Before the invention of electric light, people went to bed when it was dark and slept around for around nine hours until dawn. Even in 1960 we were sleeping for between 8 and 8.9 hours a night[5] whereas now most people get only between 6.9 and 7 hours' sleep,[6] cramming TV, shopping, Internet surfing into the night-time hours. We are all under enormous pressure to do as much as possible. We are identified and judged by our achievements and our 'busyness'. Not surprisingly, we need to stay up later and later in order to fit it all in.

Scientists have looked at cortisol levels in saliva samples and found that when people are sleep deprived the rate at which the body deals with cortisol between four and nine in the evening is six times slower than it is in people who have had enough sleep. Cortisol levels stay up too high and for too long. What's more, the ageing process appears to be increased during these hours.[7] So a lack of sleep can not only increase your levels of cortisol, making you more apple shaped, it will also make you age more quickly.

Inadequate sleep may actually cause insulin resistance too. One study looked at people who only managed to get four hours' sleep a night over six nights. They reported that the pattern of insulin and glucose was nearly identical to that which one would expect in patients with Type 2 diabetes.[8] In 2001, at the Annual Scientific Meeting of the American Diabetes Association, evidence was presented showing that people who slept for less than 6.5 hours per night (compared to 7.5–8.5 hours) released 50 per cent more insulin and were 40 per cent less sensitive to its effects.

If you are well rested, you will be much better equipped – both emotionally and physically – to cope with the demands of a busy life. Not getting enough sleep lowers your immune response. A recent study showed that missing even a few hours a night on a regular basis can decrease the number of 'natural killer cells', which are responsible for fighting off invaders such as bacteria and viruses.[9] This will come as no surprise to those of us who succumb to colds

• SLEEP MORE TO LOSE WEIGHT •

It is possible to lose weight by spending just one extra hour a night in bed! Leptin, a chemical released during sleep, suppresses the production of fat cells by curbing appetite. Leptin helps to control feelings of fullness, but when sleep is restricted leptin levels are reduced.

A study involving 500 adults aged between twenty-seven and forty over a thirteen-year period showed that in those women who put on an average of 2.25kg (5lb) in weight, their sleep fell from 7.7 to 7.3 hours per night. Those that put on the most weight slept for fewer than six hours a night.[10] Unfortunately, the longer you stay up the more likely you are to eat and low levels of leptin increase the urge. Other research has shown that leptin levels can be severely reduced by restricting sleep over just six days, so it does not take long for this effect to kick in.[11]

In one clinical trial where the volunteers' sleep was restricted, their leptin levels went down and their desire for carbohydrates (sugary foods) increased by a massive 45 per cent. It was as if their bodies were so tired they needed the sweet foods to keep them awake.[12]

If you get fewer than eight hours' sleep a night then you will end up with a higher level of body fat and a higher BMI.[13]

and other illnesses when we are 'run down' – normally after periods of insufficient sleep.

There are two main types of sleep problem: difficulty in getting off to sleep when you go to bed; and falling off to sleep easily but waking up in the middle of the night and finding it difficult to get back to sleep again.

Our physical and mental states are so intertwined that they constantly feed off one another. If something is worrying you, your body can become tense and find it hard to let go and relax. This makes sleep more elusive, which, of course, makes you feel more stressed. You worry that you are not sleeping, and are concerned about how you will cope the following day. And if you are experiencing physical symptoms, such as aches and pains, this too can make you worried and agitated, causing more tension and feelings of stress. And, not surprisingly, sleep suffers too. It's yet another vicious circle.

Tips for a good night's sleep

- Follow the dietary recommendations in Chapter 4 and especially avoid any foods or drinks containing caffeine such as tea, coffee, coke and chocolate during the day. Even decaffeinated coffee can be a problem because it contains other stimulants that can keep you awake.

- Make sure that you are eating little and often during the day to keep your blood sugar steady. This will ensure that your adrenaline levels are steady and will help to prevent the adrenal glands from overworking. This in turn means that the hormone cortisol starts to wind down when you go to bed, as it is supposed to do.
- If you regularly wake in the middle of the night – especially if you wake abruptly and with palpitations – have a small snack of complex carbohydrates, such as an oatcake or half a slice of rye bread, about an hour before bed. This will prevent your blood sugar from dropping during the night, and prevent adrenaline from being released into the bloodstream to try to correct the imbalance (known as nocturnal hypoglycaemia).
- Avoid alcohol. Not only does it affect blood sugar levels, causing adrenaline and cortisol to be released, but it also blocks the transport of tryptophan into the brain. Tryptophan is important because it is converted into serotonin, the calming and relaxing neurotransmitter.
- Have a cup of camomile tea before bed to encourage relaxation.
- Try to exercise early in the day. Exercise can be enormously stimulating, and some women find it difficult to sleep following a late workout session.
- Try using aromatherapy oils such as bergamot, lavender, roman camomile and marjoram in a warm bath, just before bed. Avoid a hot bath, which can be stimulating, but ensure that it's warm enough to encourage relaxation. A few drops of an aromatherapy oil such as lavender on your pillow at bedtime, or used in a vaporiser, can have the same effect. A pre-bed, gentle massage with the same oils will help to encourage sleep. Geranium and rosemary are particularly good for the adrenal glands.
- Keep to a sleep routine, if possible setting your alarm to wake you up at the same time each day, regardless of what time you finally fall asleep. It is also a good idea to try to be in bed by ten o'clock. It is not easy, but it does help your natural biorhythm and aids in the reduction of cortisol.
- At least an hour before bed, write yourself a 'to do' list for the next day so that you do not end up mulling over what needs to be done as you are trying to fall asleep.
- Sex can help you to get to sleep by relaxing you and releasing tension.
- Try the herbal supplements valerian, passionflower and skullcap. All these work as gentle sedatives and can help you to overcome insomnia. Try not to rely on only one herb to ensure that you don't become overly dependent. Camomile is another useful sedative, and it helps to calm and tone the nervous system, promoting restful sleep.
- Magnesium, which is known as 'Nature's tranquilliser', is good for helping with sleep problems. If you suffer from restless legs or cramps,

ensure that you are taking both magnesium and vitamin E as part of your supplementation programme.

- Use visualisation techniques. Imagine yourself on a beautiful beach with the warm sun on your skin, soft sand under your feet, blue sky, clear water and the fragrant scent of beautiful flowers. You could also have soothing music playing whilst you let yourself go and imagine yourself in this tropical paradise. This technique is very useful if you have an active mind that simply won't switch off, even when you are physically tired. By focusing the mind on something relaxing, it is much easier for it 'to let go'.
- Practise relaxation techniques (see page 115). You could try doing these with some relaxing music playing in the background.

SLEEPING PILLS

It is better to avoid sleeping pills as they alter the natural cycle of sleep during the night. During the first two thirds of the night, both deep and light sleep occur. In the last third of the night, we experience light sleep only. REM (rapid-eye movement) sleep or 'dream' sleep occurs approximately every ninety minutes. All these stages are equally important, and sleeping pills disrupt the cycle.

If you are taking pills, however, do not try to stop suddenly – you must see your doctor before cutting back.

NAPPING

It is said that both Winston Churchill and Margaret Thatcher survived on small amounts of sleep at night because they took naps during the day. Some women find that this works very well, and that a short ten- to fifteen-minute cat nap (or 'power nap') can relieve stress and renew energy.

Some women, however, claim that they feel worse after napping, or find that they simply cannot sleep for short periods of time, and end up losing an hour or so a day in an attempt to get a short, refreshing rest.

The trick in napping is to fall asleep sitting up. If you go to bed or lie down the tendency is to go into a deeper sleep, which makes you feel groggy if you do not get enough, or it sends you off to sleep for too long. The optimum length of time for a nap is between twenty-five and thirty minutes.

• Chapter 8 •

It's All in Your Genes

How your genes can tell you the best diet for you

Can your genetic make-up affect your body shape? And can your genes dictate the diet that is best for you? The answer to both of these questions is yes. Through genetic testing you can learn whether you need to eat a low-fat diet or just cut down on food generally; whether a glass of wine is actually beneficial for you given your genetic make-up or whether it should be left well alone; whether you should be eating more cabbage or taking supplements, and if so which. The answers are all in your genes.

For clues about the effects of genes on diet, body shape and weight, scientists have studied our ancestors and their lifestyles. Our hormone systems today are very similar to those of our ancestors even though they had to forage for nuts and berries, hunt down and kill their dinner and, in times of scarcity, go hungry. We today need hunt no further than the nearest supermarket where we can find our meat not just placated, but skinned, sliced and wrapped in plastic and in a quantity determined only by our funds! Our food may have evolved into a selection of processed, refined carbohydrates, saturated fats and sugars that our ancestors certainly would not recognise. Yet our genetic make-up really hasn't changed.

In days gone by those people with the slowest metabolisms were the most likely to survive times without food because their bodies worked efficiently to save everything possible as fat, only burning what was absolutely necessary for energy. Their 'efficient' metabolism kept them alive. Survivors would have carried a gene that allowed them to store any excess calories as fat – an energy store for emergencies. Even today, in certain cultures, where food supply varies noticeably with the seasons, people have the ability to create energy stores and their body weight can vary dramatically.[1] In modern Western society, a person with that kind of genetic make-up is not regarded as quite so fortunate. They are the ones who must watch what they eat or else they will put on weight.

So when food is scarce, a slow metabolism gives you an advantage but in our society of plentiful, cheap, fast food, it represents a distinct health disadvantage.

THE 'THRIFTY GENE'

But genes are not the only factor in this particular equation. As obesity expert Dr George Bray said, 'Genetics load the gun, environment pulls the trigger.' The Pima, Native Americans of southern Arizona, have what is called a 'thrifty gene'. Their metabolism is very efficiently geared to accumulating fat in preparation for times of famine.

For over two thousand years the Pima Indians grew wheat, beans and pumpkins. At the end of the nineteenth century, however, their water supply was diverted by Western settlers. In order to survive they ate the food given to them by the US government which included white flour and sugar. Over time their diet has become increasingly processed and typically American and this has clashed badly with their metabolism; thanks to their 'thrifty genotype', they are now the fattest people on earth with nine out of every ten being overweight or obese. Most of them are insulin resistant by the age of eight and children as young as three develop Type 2 diabetes. Although they are eating the same junk as the rest of the population their diabetes rate has soared to the point where it is ten times higher than in their Caucasian counterparts.

So although we all live within the constraints of our genetic make-up, what we eat and how we live really can shape the action of those genes.

It is thought that some of us can have a genetic predisposition to store fat around the middle and become apple shaped.[2] These genetic factors could, on average, give someone a lower metabolic rate, a tendency to have higher insulin levels and a greater likelihood of being insulin resistant. But the lead researcher on one of the gene studies looking at fat around the middle adds: 'If you control your diet and exercise often, in most cases you can override the effects of this genetic burden. You may have to try a little harder, but chances are that, with lifestyle interventions, you can control the obesity' (endocrinologist Alan Shuldiner, M.D. of the Division of Geriatric Medicine and Gerontology at Johns Hopkins Bayview Medical Centre, Maryland in America).

So a genetic predisposition does not mean that you are 'stuck' with that weight around the middle. You might just have to work a bit harder than a friend of yours who can eat anything and stay slim.

NATURE VS NURTURE

In August 2000, the Office of Genetics and Disease Prevention in America issued a statement (the Gene-Environment Interaction Fact Sheet) saying:

> Virtually all human diseases result from the interaction of genetic susceptibility and modifiable environmental factors, broadly defined to include infectious, chemical, physical, nutritional and behavioural factors. Variations in genetic make-up are associated with almost all disease.

Genetic variations do not cause disease but rather influence a person's susceptibility to environmental factors.

Genetic information can be used to target interventions.

What this means, for the purposes of this book, is that we each have a unique set of genes that can make us more susceptible to producing more cortisol, more insulin and more fat around the middle.[3] But understanding the workings of these unique genes can help us to make the diet and lifestyle changes (what the scientists call our 'environment', basically anything that is not genetic) that can reduce our risk of developing these problems. Rather than forcing us to accept life with the spectre of a predetermined disease hanging over us, our genes give us important information that we can use to our advantage.

Some people can get away with being a couch potato because of their genes whilst others cannot. A study of twenty-eight pairs of identical male twins (identical twins share the same genetic make-up) was undertaken, looking at the impact of lifestyle on genes (where one brother was a self-confessed couch potato, whilst his twin was a long-distance runner, for example). For six weeks the twins were given a high-fat diet, followed by six weeks on a low-fat diet. At the end of each six-week period, their cholesterol levels were measured. Despite their hugely different lifestyles, each pair of twins reacted similarly to the change in diet. Their genetic make-up completely dominated the proceedings. Researchers replicated the study on other twins and found that some pairs were very sensitive to the high-fat diet whilst others showed no changes in cholesterol no matter how much they ate or exercised. But in all cases, both twins in every pair responded in the same way. As Paul Williams, the lead researcher, said, 'Our experiment shows how important our genes are. Some people have to be careful about their diets while others have more freedom.'[4]

USING GENETIC INFORMATION

The important point about genetic tests is that they give you information. Think about life and genetic testing in terms of a game of cards. You will be dealt some cards that cannot be changed and you will be stuck with these for the whole game (your eye colour, for example). Then there are others, like the 'thrifty gene', which you might not have chosen, but which could be useful depending on how you play them. But what if you were not allowed to look at the hand you had been dealt? You would have very little chance of winning.

Conventional medicine tends to be very 'anti'-based: antibiotic, anti-inflammatory, antihistamine and antidepressants. Its focus is often on treating the symptoms rather than the underlying cause so that when, for example, anti-inflammatory drugs are stopped the painful joints return because the drugs were not addressing the reason why the joints were painful in the first place.

The preventative medicine that I advocate is, I feel, the medicine of the future and predictive genetics testing will play a large part in that. It will also be used increasingly in conventional medicine so that it can evolve from a one-size-fits-all approach to finding the right drug for the right person at the right time.

This field of science is termed 'pharmacogenetics'. It uses genetic information to fine-tune the right drug to the right person. In June 2004, the British government announced a £50 million investment in making the NHS 'a world leader in genetics-based healthcare'. It is a huge area of research and development for the future. The UK BioBank, involving half a million people, is a study of genes, environment and health aimed to be delivered in ten years' time to identify the major genetic and environmental factors that contribute to disease.

This is the future of medicine, and that includes nutritional medicine, so that we will be able to match the right diet and supplements programme with the right person. As the eighteenth-century physician Caleb Parry said, 'It is much more important to know what kind of patient has a disease than to know what kind of disease a patient has.'

Genetic tests are currently available that can give us information as to what diet (way of eating) is best for any individual. The results can pinpoint foods that are best avoided, foods they should eat more of and supplements that would be especially useful for them because of their genetic make-up.

(For more information on these genetic tests see my clinic contact details in Resources, page 183.)

• Chapter 9 •

TESTING, TESTING

The tests which pinpoint your fat-making triggers

You may have absolutely no doubt that you carry your fat around the middle of your body; the fat distribution will be obvious. Likewise, you'll have a pretty good idea when the recommendations in this book start working because your body shape will fundamentally change. And, along with your changing silhouette, the dangerous health implications of being apple shaped will also diminish.

For many people that is enough.

Others, however, like to see their problem in black and white (preferably on graph paper) and to see the physiological evidence that proves that what they are doing is helping to correct that problem. This is where laboratory tests come in.

I believe that lab tests should be used regularly, in much the same way that we do MOT tests on our cars to pinpoint problems before they get out of hand. It is always worth knowing that your brake pads are wearing thin and need to be replaced before the brakes actually fail, causing a serious accident. The same applies to your body, the vehicle that will carry you through life. Naturally you want it to function as well as it can for as long as it can. So imagine the value of being able to pick up a potential problem before it occurs, and then reversing that problem.

There are a number of tests that I think are very useful in the diagnosis and treatment of fat around the middle. The health implications I laid out in Chapter 3 make it quite clear that this can become far more than just a cosmetic problem, or the inconvenience of ill-fitting clothes. Wouldn't it be useful for you to know whether your tummy fat is causing changes to take place within your body that could signal the start of serious health problems? This would give you the opportunity to take stock and follow the recommendations in this book wholeheartedly for the sake of your future health.

I would therefore recommend the following basic tests:

- Adrenal stress test
- Insulin resistance test
- Food allergy test
- Yeasts and parasite test

Let's now take a detailed look at these tests.

ADRENAL STRESS TEST

The best way to know for sure whether or not you have elevated cortisol levels is with an adrenal stress test.

Blood tests are not particularly helpful for this purpose as they are designed to pick up severe adrenal diseases such as Cushing's syndrome (in which cortisol is too high) and Addison's disease (cortisol is too low). They are not very helpful when we are looking for something more subtle.

Furthermore, cortisol fluctuates during the day, ideally being highest in the morning and lowest at night when you are ready to wind down and go to bed (see diagram below). It is most useful to look at this pattern of cortisol over a twenty-four-hour period to see whether it stays within the normal range throughout the day.

Pattern of cortisol over a 24-hour period

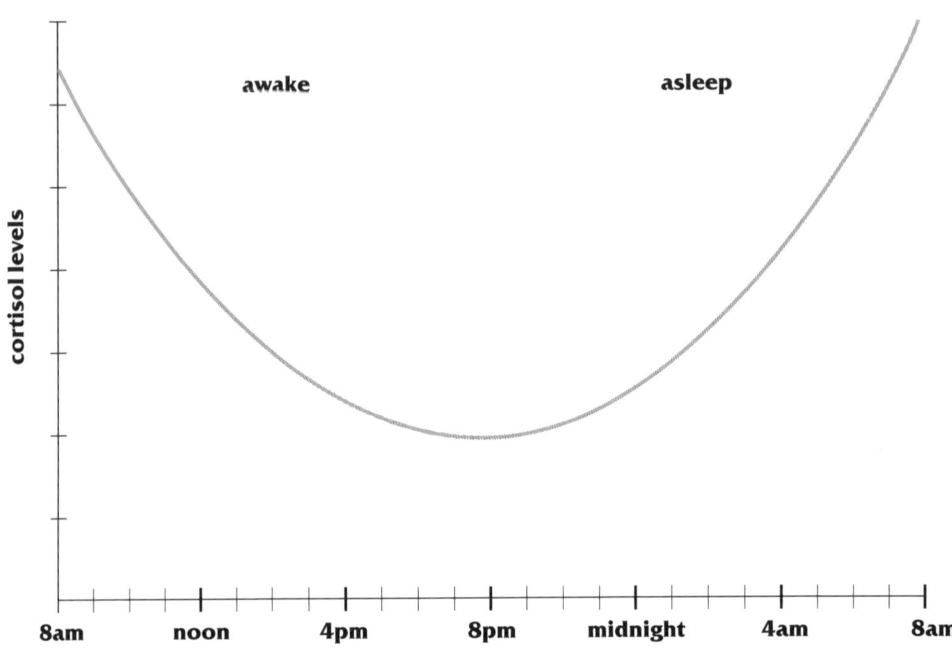

How is the test done?

Because blood tests would need to be taken four times a day in order to get a true picture, the test is done using your saliva instead. Four saliva samples are collected in a kit at home over the course of a day and the samples are then sent back to the lab for analysis. The test also measures your DHEA (dehydroepiandrosterone), the hormone that works to balance many of the negative effects of cortisol and helps you to cope with stress. Research has shown that DHEA helps to improve memory function, boost energy levels, and has an anti-weight effect by decreasing fat tissue, excess insulin and food intake. Most importantly, DHEA appears to protect the immune system from some of the cell damage caused by ageing and disease. So it is important to have good levels of DHEA and this can be checked in the adrenal stress test.

Scientists have looked at the association between fat around the middle and cortisol levels measured in saliva. They have found that high levels of cortisol measured in a sample taken first thing in the morning after waking correlated significantly with fat around the middle of the body.[1]

In addition to being a good indicator for fat around the middle, you might be interested in other research into cortisol levels and women's health just to see how far-reaching the effect can be and why it is important to control high cortisol for reasons other than just looking good. Research is now looking into whether the diurnal (daily) rhythm of cortisol can be used to predict breast cancer survival, as it is known that cortisol affects the immune system and the ability of natural killer cells to do their job effectively.[2] In one study cortisol levels over a day were shown to be a valid predictor of subsequent survival up to seven years later[3] and other research is looking into differences between women with and without breast cancer in relation to their diurnal cortisol rhythms.[4]

My advice is to take this test, if possible, before following the recommendations in this book, then re-testing three months later to help you see the difference.

(For more information on this test see Resources, page 183.)

INSULIN RESISTANCE TEST

It is useful to know whether you are already insulin resistant because if you are you should pay particular attention to the dietary recommendations in Chapter 4. The condition is reversible if caught soon enough.

As we already know fat around your middle is one sign of insulin resistance. Another is extreme blood sugar peaks and troughs during the day. Unfortunately, these can progress to Type 2 diabetes (late onset diabetes) if left unchecked so it is much better to prevent a problem like this than to wait and then deal with it once it has occurred.

How is the test done?

To measure insulin resistance, a simple glucose test is not enough; insulin levels should be tested too as with insulin resistance both glucose and insulin levels can be high.

The insulin resistance test is a fasting blood test, which means that your blood is taken first thing in the morning before you have eaten or drunk anything. You can use a kit which you can then take to your local practice nurse or doctor so that they can send it away to the lab. The results are forwarded on to you with an accompanying explanation. The blood test also measures cholesterol, HDL ('good') cholesterol, LDL ('bad') cholesterol, triglycerides and VDL (very low-density lipoproteins) because these can be outside the normal ranges with insulin resistance. High levels of LDL and VDL can increase the risk of atherosclerosis (a build-up of plaque on the artery walls). An analysis of the results of a huge study across fifty-two countries in 2004 showed that 45 per cent of heart attacks are caused by having abnormal cholesterol and lipid (fat) levels.[5] However the study does make the important point that these are 'modifiable risk factors' which means that something can be done to reduce the risk.

(For more information on this test see Resources, page 183.)

Note: if you are getting symptoms of excessive thirst and are urinating frequently it is important to consult your doctor in order to check for diabetes.

FOOD ALLERGY TEST

There are two types of food allergy. A classic allergy is one that is apparent immediately after someone has eaten (or, sometimes, just come into contact with) a food to which they are allergic (peanuts, for instance). Their blood would show raised levels of IgE antibodies and in extreme cases this type of allergy can cause anaphylactic shock and can be fatal. This is an abnormal immunological reaction to food and it is crucial that the person knows which foods are causing it so that they can avoid them in the future.

The other type of allergy, more often called intolerance, is not so striking and is harder to detect, yet it still involves the immune system. Most allergic reactions of this type stimulate the release of histamine and other substances that produce inflammation.

We saw in Chapter 3 that your fat cells can produce substances called inflammatory cytokines, which have the effect of pumping up the immune system so that the adrenal glands then release more cortisol to calm it down. The excess cortisol causes more fat storage which then releases more inflammatory cytokines. Yes, it's another vicious circle. The cytokines also prevent the binding of insulin on to the receptors, so increasing your likelihood of insulin resistance.

Cortisol is a strong anti-inflammatory which is quite naturally called into play when you have an allergic reaction to a particular food. So by eating foods that your body finds it difficult to deal with, you are actually causing a rise in cortisol and reinforcing the message to store fat. This is why so many people report a dramatic loss of weight when they eliminate from their diet foods to which they are allergic.

Over time, the release of histamine and other inflammatory substances will alter the permeability of the gut making it 'leaky' so that food molecules escape into the bloodstream. This then sets off an immune response because the body treats these food particles as foreign substances and starts to attack them. This is how you can become allergic to substances that previously gave you no problems at all.

If you have any of the following symptoms as well as fat around your middle then it worth considering a Food Allergy Test so that you can establish which foods and drinks do not suit you:

- bloating
- excess wind (flatulence)
- diarrhoea
- constipation
- chronic infections
- skin problems such as itching, rashes, eczema etc.
- fatigue
- joint and muscle pains
- arthritis
- headaches/migraines
- rhinitis (constant runny nose)
- sinus problems

How is the test done?

The test measures your reaction to 233 different foods, seasonings, colourings, additives and drinks from one single blood sample. As with the insulin resistance test you will be sent a kit that you can then take to your practice nurse or doctor. A sample of blood can then be posted back to the laboratory for analysis.

(For more information on this test see Resources, page 183.)

YEAST AND PARASITE TEST

Unfortunately, yeasts and parasites in the digestive system also cause an immune response and cytokines will be released to deal with them.

Persistent vaginal thrush can be one of the symptoms of candidiasis, but other symptoms can include:

- food cravings, especially for sugar and bread
- fatigue
- a bloated stomach with excess flatulence
- a feeling of being 'spaced out'
- becoming tipsy on a very small amount of alcohol.

Symptoms of a parasitic infection include:

- irritable bowel syndrome
- bloating
- constipation
- loose stools
- feeling full, especially after eating
- belching after meals
- indigestion
- wind (flatulence/gas)
- bowels not being 'right' since an episode of food poisoning
- abdominal cramps

Both yeasts and parasites can cause bloating – this can sometimes be so severe as to make some people look seven months pregnant and feel much fatter around the middle than they actually are. So it is important to know for sure what is actually happening in your body.

As you can see some of the symptoms of yeasts and parasites overlap so it is useful to do a test that combines them both. Of course, you should always see your doctor first if you are getting physical symptoms but if you have been given the all clear medically it is worth looking for another cause.

How is the test done?

Yeasts and parasites are tested for using a stool sample collected at home and then sent back to the laboratory in the kit provided. The results will tell you whether you have a yeast, like candida, or parasites, which ones they are and what you need to do about them.

(For more information on this test see Resources, page 183.)

Although I have talked about four tests in this chapter the two most important in terms of fat around the middle are the adrenal stress test and the insulin resistance test because they are so directly related to the problem you are hoping to solve.

I recommend doing these two tests first, before you do anything else, so that you know just what your starting point is. Then follow the recommendations in this book for three months and see what happens to your general health. As you change your lifestyle and put in place the dietary recommendations from Chapter 4 you may find that some other symptoms that seemed completely unrelated to being apple shaped will start to improve. You may then need to do a test for food allergies, yeasts or parasites if you notice lingering symptoms that are just not shifting, but you may not.

• Chapter 10 •

THE 'LOSE-YOUR-BELLY' (AND 'FIND-YOUR-WAIST') PLAN OF ACTION

This is your 'Do it!' chapter, your personal plan of action and you should stick to it as closely as you can for the next three months. Although you can simply start here, I would really recommend that you have a read through the rest of the book first, to gain a little understanding about the 'science' of how and why fat accumulates around the middle of your body. Once you have had a chance to take all that on board, and you are – I hope – sufficiently convinced that something can be done, you can make a start on the plan.

The results you will see on this programme will be more striking if you undertake all aspects of it, so only start when you're really ready and thoroughly committed. You will need to put in a bit of effort at first until you are familiar with the right foods to buy, the supplements to take and the exercise and lifestyle regimes, but it will swiftly become familiar. It's like learning to drive a car. There's a lot to think about at first (speed, changing gears, indicating, looking in the mirror) but before long it all becomes completely automatic and you perform all those separate functions without even thinking. Once you are in the routine it will be effortless. And it's only for three months of your life – which is not such a long time when you consider the enormous long-term benefits not only in terms of looking good, but also your future health. After this period of time you can then ease up and reintroduce some of the foods and drink that you left out (see the maintenance plan in Chapter 11).

So, to make this 'lose-your-belly' (and 'find-your-waist'!) plan really effective you should tackle all four elements at once:

- Nutrition
- Supplements
- Exercise
- Lifestyle

GETTING STARTED

My advice is to ditch the scales. Muscle weighs three times as much as fat so you can be losing fat but not see it on the scales. Because fat takes up five times as much space as muscle, your body will be changing shape as you lose fat and gain muscle and the best way to see and record that fat loss is by measuring yourself.

So, before you do anything else, get a tape measure and take the following measurements now:

Place A: just under your bust where your bra goes
Place B: around your waist above your navel
Place C: over the largest bit of your fat around the middle

Write the measurements in the table below and repeat this every four weeks over the next three months.

	1st month **Date:**	**2nd month** **Date:**	**3rd month** **Date:**
Place A			
Place B			
Place C			

If you have fat percentage scales (or if you have access to some at your local gym) you can add a column for your fat percentage reading every four weeks.

NUTRITION

This is the 'How to eat' section. It's not a diet, merely your new healthy eating programme for the next three months. Aim to stick to the eating plan at least 80 per cent of the time and allow yourself 20 per cent off for good behaviour (and human fallibility!). Nobody's perfect and you simply will not be able to eat right 100 per cent of the time, so don't beat yourself up about it or feel guilty. Worse still, do not resort to the classic dieter's reaction, namely, 'I've blown it now so I might as well have a whole packet of biscuits and start again another day.' One biscuit once in a while will not ruin everything. Just follow the recommendations most of the time and do your best when you go out, or on holiday or to parties (see my tips on page 156).

There are a number of key strategies that make the nutrition part of this plan work. I call them my 'Oh-so-simple nine-step eating plan' and this is described in detail on pages 53–82. In this chapter we will focus more on how to implement the plan, starting with when to eat.

When to eat

Eat every three hours. This stops your body from thinking it is starving (a stress), reduces cortisol (so it won't store more fat), boosts your metabolism (food is plentiful so the body does not need to store it) and stops cravings and binges (blood sugar has not dropped because you are keeping it topped up). Because you are eating regularly you will not feel hungry and so your appetite is under control. The end result is that you burn up fat and the best news of all is that the fat around your middle will be the first to go.

To help shift the weight around your middle as efficiently as possible avoid eating starchy carbohydrates after six o'clock in the evening (no rice, potatoes or pasta – not even brown rice and wholemeal pasta).

• KEY EATING STRATEGIES •

- Eat three main meals, but make them smaller than you would normally.
- Eat a mid-morning snack and a mid-afternoon snack.
- No starchy carbohydrates after six in the evening.

Tip: if you wake up with low blood sugar in the morning, or during the night (your heart may be pounding and you may be unable to get back to sleep) it is very likely that your blood sugar level has dropped overnight and adrenaline has kicked in. Eating a small, starchy snack (an oatcake, for example) an hour before going to bed will help to alleviate these symptoms until you have totally mastered the art of getting your blood sugar under control during the day.

WHAT TO EAT

(and what not to eat)

Photocopy this page and stick it on your cupboard door

- Include protein (vegetable or animal) with every meal
- Swap from refined carbohydrates (white flour, white rice, pasta) to whole carbohydrates (rye, oats, brown rice, corn pasta, quinoa)
- Reduce consumption of potatoes and sweet potatoes
- Eliminate sugar and honey
- Change from tea, coffee, colas to mineral water, herb teas or grain coffee (from health-food stores)
- Reduce saturated fat and include foods containing essential fatty acids (oily fish, nuts and seeds)
- Add spices to your food such as cloves, turmeric, cinnamon and bay leaves as these are known to have a positive effect on insulin. Try sprinkling cinnamon on your porridge in the mornings.
- Eliminate soft fizzy drinks
- Avoid foods and drinks that contain artificial sweeteners
- Avoid bananas, grapes for the first three months
- Avoid fruit juice (unless very diluted)
- Stay away from foods that are labelled low fat, low calorie or 'diet'
- Reduce your intake of red meat, chicken and cow's dairy products (milk, cream, cheese)
- Use organic live plain yogurts as the dairy food of choice and in moderation sheep's and goat's cheese
- Eat more fish and eggs
- Eat more beans (lentils, kidney beans, chick peas etc.) and organic soya products
- Eat more nuts, seeds, avocados
- Eliminate margarines and use (sparingly) organic butter instead
- Eliminate alcohol, or, at least, dramatically reduce consumption and stick to wine or spirits NOT beer

SHOPPING LIST

On pages 141–155 there are some meal and snack suggestions but in addition to this I want to show you the huge choice of foods that is available to you – this plan really does not have to be restrictive at all. Take this list with you when you go shopping before you start the plan so that you can stock up on a good variety of foods and have lots to choose from. Some of these foods probably won't be available at smaller supermarkets, so try to stock up at a really big store or try looking in your local health-food shop.

Nuts – brazils, almonds, cashews, pistachio, peanuts

Seeds – sunflower, sesame, linseeds (flax), pumpkin

Beans – soya, kidney, aduki, butter, chick peas and haricot (if you buy baked beans look for no-sugar, no-sweetener brands)

Fish – oily fish (sardines, mackerel, tuna (tinned tuna does not contain much Omega 3 but fresh does), salmon, swordfish, herring (including kippers), white fish (cod, haddock, plaice, sole), shellfish (but watch the amount of shellfish you eat if your cholesterol is already high)

Eggs – buy organic free range.

Dairy – organic live plain yogurt, sparingly cottage cheese, feta cheese and other sheep and goat's cheese. Use rice, oat and organic soya milk as alternatives to dairy.

Grains – brown rice, oats, rye, quinoa (actually a seed but used like a grain), buckwheat (actually part of the rhubarb family but used like a grain), millet, barley, maize, wholewheat (but you will feel less bloated without wheat as it is so difficult to digest)

Vegetables – broccoli, cabbage, celery, cauliflower, Brussels sprouts, asparagus, leeks, onions, green beans, squash, cucumber, tomatoes, mushrooms, courgettes, radish, spring greens, swedes, turnips, kale, lettuce, carrots, beetroots, etc. Stock up on frozen vegetables too.

Fruit – apples, pears, blackberries, cherries, raspberries, blueberries, plums, peaches, oranges, kiwi, clementines, satsumas, melon, watermelon, pineapple

Seaweed – Look for nori flakes in your health-food shop. They are mineral rich and can be sprinkled on rice or vegetables.

Prepared foods – soups in jars and cans (buy organic where possible and avoid those with sugar or artificial sweeteners – instant miso soup (sold in supermarkets and health-food shops) is a good standby for lunch), pasta sauces (no sugar), hummus (organic if possible), tofu and smoked tofu, breakfast cereals (unsweetened or sweetened with apple juice rather than sugar). Sugar-free (and sweetener-free) jam. Fill your store cupboard with tins of organic beans (kidney, butter etc.) to use as instant protein and excellent fibre to add to salads, casseroles or stir-fries.

Snack foods – in a really good health-food shop you will find fruit bars and other snacks which do not have added sugar.

Drinks – herbal teas like peppermint, camomile, redbush (Rooibos – South African tea that grows naturally without caffeine), grain coffees, pure fruit juices but only very diluted for the first three months, sparkling mineral water and this can be added to fruit juice. Avoid fruit teas for the first three months and any tea which says 'flavouring' in the ingredient list.

• BREAKFAST – SOME DOS AND DON'TS •

• Porridge oats: get organic where possible and cook with water. (Do not buy the quick or instant porridge because its speed of cooking means that it is absorbed into the bloodstream faster.) Top with ground flaxseeds (linseeds) (you can buy them ready ground at health-food shops or grind them yourself in a blender), a mix of seeds like sesame, sunflower and pumpkin, or sliced, blanched or whole almonds. You could also add some berries to sweeten it or a spoonful of sugar-free jam (pure fruit jam not diabetic jam, from health-food shops).

• Grilled kippers, sardines, herring or mackerel fillets with grilled tomatoes and mushrooms. Avoid the artificially coloured kippers and look for browner, less red or orange, undyed kippers.

• Rye bread with sugar-free jam (pure fruit not diabetic jam, from health-food shops) or a pure nut butter (such as peanut, cashew nut or almond butter). Avoid nut butters made with palm oil as this is a saturated fat. The ideal is nuts ground into a butter with nothing else added.

• Yogurt: organic, live, plain yogurt with chopped-up pieces of fruit or blended to make a smoothie. Sprinkle with nuts and/or seeds.

• Muesli: you can buy a good sugar-free muesli from your health-food shop. Look out for wheat-free versions too. Soak the muesli in apple juice, orange juice, rice, soya or oat milk for about twenty minutes (or overnight if you like it really mushy) as this breaks down the phytates in the raw grain and means that you will get more goodness from the food. If the muesli does not already contain nuts or seeds, add this important protein to your bowl. (See also muesli recipe opposite.)

BREAKFAST – TIPS, SUGGESTIONS AND RECIPES

Never miss breakfast and **always** eat within an hour of waking in the morning.

HOMEMADE MUESLI

Serves 1

- Use raw ingredients of your choice, preferably organic wholegrain cereals, better still if wheat-free.
- 25g (1oz) of either one or a combination of oats, rice flakes, millet flakes, barley flakes, rye flakes or buckwheat flakes
- 1½ heaped tablespoons whole or freshly ground seeds (flaxseeds, pumpkin, pine kernels and/or sesame)
- ½ tablespoon whole or crushed fresh nuts (optional) (almonds, brazils, cashews, pecan and/or hazelnut)
- a good handful mixed fresh fruit (berries, kiwi, apple, etc.)
- Serve with 200ml (7fl oz) oat milk, rice milk, or organic soya milk and a tablespoon of goat's, sheep's or organic live plain yogurt if desired.

PROTEIN KICK-START

Serves 1

Blend the following:

- 150g (5½oz) frozen mixed berries (strawberries, blueberries, raspberries, blackcurrants, blackberries) or other fruit of choice
- (½ banana – only after the first three months)
- 150ml (5fl oz) rice, oat or soya milk or water
- 150–175ml (5–6fl oz) filtered water
- 1 heaped tablespoon ground almonds and seeds (sesame, pumpkin, flaxseeds, pine kernels)
- 1 tablespoon flaxseed (linseed) oil

Scrambled, Poached or Boiled Egg

- Serve with one slice of rye or pumpernickel bread, an oatcake or a rice, buckwheat or wheat-free cracker. Garnish with tomato and fresh herbs.

Breakfast Omelettes

Serves 1

- Beat together 2 eggs with 2 tablespoons non-dairy milk.
- Heat a small teaspoon of organic olive oil in a small frying pan and pour in the egg mixture. Carefully stir the eggs to fold the mixture.
- When nearly set, add a filling of tomato, onion, red pepper or leftover vegetables from last night's dinner with a sprinkling of dried herbs.

Berry Booster

Serves 1

Blend the following:

- 250g (9oz) pot natural, plain, organic, live yogurt
- 2 tablespoons mixed berries
- 1 tablespoon ground mixed seeds/nuts
- 1 tablespoon flaxseed (linseed) oil

No-sugar, Organic Baked Beans

- Serve on rye bread or other wheat-free option.

SUGGESTIONS FOR LUNCHES

Smoked mackerel and salad

Leftover stir-fry from the night before, with brown rice

Hummus and vegetables tucked into wholemeal pitta bread (only use the pitta after your first four weeks)

Instant miso soups – available from health-food shops – with a bean salad

Tuna fish and brown rice salad

Pasta made from corn (available in supermarkets and health-food shops) with tuna or beans

Guacamole with raw vegetable sticks or oatcakes

Curried brown rice with vegetables and nuts

Quinoa with stir-fried vegetables

Smoked salmon or smoked salmon pâté with salad

Grilled sardines on rye bread

Sardines (tinned) on rye bread toast topped with tomatoes

• LUNCH – SOME DOS AND DON'TS •

Try to have a palm-sized amount of protein with lunch and no more than half a palm-sized amount of starchy carbohydrates such as brown rice or corn or vegetable pasta and one or two palm-sized portions of raw or cooked vegetables.

Soups: always have a protein, so choose a fish or bean soup with a slice of rye bread or oatcakes; carrot and cashew nut soup is another delicious option.

DINNER

SALADS

Start with a base of salad vegetables, such as lettuce, cucumber, tomato and spring onion, then add any of the following:

- avocado, red grapefruit, grated ginger and caraway seeds
- beansprouts and sweetcorn
- apple, celery, beans and chopped walnuts
- red kidney beans, sweetcorn and green beans
- avocado, tofu and pineapple
- beetroot, pineapple, pitted prunes, chopped walnuts and lemon juice
- grated carrot, sultanas, orange and pumpkin seeds with honey and mustard dressing
- cooked brown rice, sweetcorn and kidney beans with herbs
- cooked brown rice, grated carrot, diced celery, sliced radish and sunflower seeds
- poached salmon, capers and lemon juice
- tuna, celery and cooked brown rice
- tuna, mixed beans, orange, cashew nuts and French dressing
- cooked millet, red pepper, celery, chopped mint, chives and parsley
- red cabbage, onion, apple, raisins with lemon or orange juice

• DINNER – SOME DOS AND DON'TS •

Avoid starchy carbohydrates at this meal if you can until you have lost the weight around the middle. Have a palm-size portion of protein with two palm-sized portions of raw or cooked vegetables. Vary the vegetables so that your meals are interesting and vary the cooking methods too – try steaming, roasting and stir-frying (in olive oil). Use herbs and spices (garlic, lemongrass, ginger, tamari, lemon, miso, turmeric, cinnamon, etc.) for different flavours.

SALAD DRESSINGS

Avoid commercial dressings as they usually contain sugar. It's much cheaper (and healthier) to make your own.

Simple French dressing: mix together well 4 tablespoons olive oil, 4 tablespoons lemon juice, a pinch of dried herbs and 1 clove fresh garlic.

Tofu mayonnaise: process together 1 x 275g (10oz) packet organic tofu, 1 tablespoon lemon juice, 1/2 teaspoon mustard powder. Slowly add 200ml (7fl oz) oil (use a mixture of olive and sunflower) and process on full power. Store the mayonnaise in the fridge, in a covered container. Flavour with garlic, herbs, onions or sugar-free tomato purée.

Yogurt dressing: add a few herbs or diced cucumber and chopped mint to natural, organic bio yogurt.

Tofu and lemon dressing: blend 1 x 275g (10oz) packet tofu with 2 tablespoons fresh lemon juice, 2 tablespoons olive oil and 1 clove garlic or fresh chives.

Avocado dressing: blend together juice of 1 lemon, 1 large avocado, salt and pepper. Add olive oil and/or soya milk until you get the consistency you want.

HOT MEALS

Steam stir-fry vegetables with tofu and toasted cashews

Vegetable and bean risotto

Bean, vegetable and tofu casserole

Stuffed peppers, aubergines, marrow or butternut squash (stuff with brown rice, pine kernels and sultanas)

Carrots, coconut and brown rice

Sushi with brown rice

Steam stir-fry prawns, spring onions and cashews with brown rice

Lentil and vegetable curry or chilli with brown rice

Grilled fish with tomato and pesto

Corn and spinach pasta or rice pasta with vegetables in a tomato sauce

Note: to steam stir-fry add both olive oil and water to the pan and cook quickly keeping the lid on to allow the food to steam. This prevents the oil from reaching very high temperatures at which the fats become damaged and can impair health.

QUICK MEALS

- 200g (7oz) tuna (drain off the oil or use tuna in spring water), 2 pilchards, 4 sardines, 225g (8oz) prawns, lentils or mixed bean salad, served with a large mixed salad of your choice. Use 1/2 tablespoon flaxseed (linseed) oil as a dressing. Serves 1.
- Two-egg (organic) omelette (mushrooms and leek, herb, garlic, tomato and grated courgette), served with a large mixed salad. Use 1/2 tablespoon flaxseed (linseed) oil as a dressing. Serves 1.
- Falafel and mixed salad on toasted pumpernickel bread.
- Warm mackerel salad (serves 1). Grill 50g (2oz) mackerel fillets for 6–7 minutes to heat through. Serve on top of a mixed salad made up of 1/2 ripe avocado, pitted, peeled and sliced, 1 ripe mango, pitted, peeled and sliced and assorted salad leaves. Top with toasted sunflower seeds (see tips section for recipe).
- Stir-fry prawns or organic tofu with a selection of stir-fried vegetables. Use 1/2 tablespoon olive oil to stir-fry. Add tamari soya sauce plus mixed herbs to taste.
- Greek salad (serves 1). Chop and mix lettuce, tomato, peppers, cucumber with olives and 110g (4oz) feta cheese cut into chunks. Serve with a yogurt dressing.
- Baked salmon or mackerel parcel (serves 1). Place 110g (4oz) salmon or mackerel fillets in a casserole dish, brush with olive oil, season with black pepper and place a slice of lemon on top. Bake for 20–30 minutes at 190°C/375°F/gas mark 5. Serve with a mixed salad.
- Tofu salad with mixed vegetable salad (serves 1). Chop and combine 25g (1oz) red cabbage, 25g (1oz) broccoli florets, 1 medium carrot, 1 stick celery, 1 spring onion with 75g (3oz) smoked or diced tofu.

Note: if you want to use tofu raw, always put it into boiling water for a few minutes (blanching) then leave to cool.

- Homemade vegetable soup with lentils or mixed beans.
- Oatcakes spread with a mackerel pâté, tofu or tuna spread.

  For the tofu spread: mix together 275g (10oz) tofu, 1 tablespoon tomato purée, 1/2 teaspoon garlic granules, a pinch of dried basil and some freshly ground black pepper until smooth.

For the tuna spread: simmer 2 large chopped carrots (or a mix of carrot and parsnip), together with a chopped onion, in a very little water until soft and the liquid has reduced to 2 tablespoons. Mash well and mix in 1 small tin of tuna (drained).

- Homemade hummus using 1 tin organic chick peas, drained and rinsed. Purée the chick peas in a blender with the juice of 2 lemons and 1 tablespoon cold-pressed olive oil. Sieve, then add 1/2–1 teaspoon fresh garlic, 110g (4oz) ground sesame seeds and 1–2 tablespoons tahini, mixing the mixture to form a thick paste. Add a little water if necessary. Keep refrigerated.
- Bean pâté with oatcakes – this is quick to make, it just takes a little preparation. Soak a handful of mixed beans overnight. Cook for 1–2 hours until soft. Drain and rinse then roughly mash with a fork. Add some chopped spring onions, crushed garlic if desired, a tablespoon of cold-pressed salad oil of your choice and a tablespoon of tahini. Organic mayonnaise may be added to taste. Sprinkle with herbs and black pepper and blend.
- Haricot beans and watercress salad.
- Wild salmon with vegetables and brown rice.
- Stir-fried vegetables with brown rice, prawns and nuts.

MAIN MEAL RECIPE SUGGESTIONS

BEAN BURGERS

Serves 4

450g (1lb) dried mixed beans (you can buy ready-mixed beans from the supermarket – often called a 'soup mix')
1 tablespoon finely chopped fresh parsley
2 teaspoons dried tarragon
1 egg, beaten
1 garlic clove, crushed
freshly ground black pepper to taste
1 tablespoon sunflower oil
1 onion, chopped

- Soak the mixed beans in cold water overnight. Place in water and bring to the boil, simmer for 2 hours.
- Preheat the oven to 180°C/350°F/gas mark 4.
- When the beans are soft, remove from the pan, drain and then place in a bowl and mash well. Add the parsley, tarragon, egg, garlic and pepper and mix well.
- Heat the oil in a frying pan and gently fry the onion for 2–3 minutes. Add the onion to the bean mixture and stir well.
- Form the mixture into round burger shapes and place on a greased baking sheet.
- Bake in the oven for 15–20 minutes or until golden brown, turning halfway through cooking. Serve with salad or steamed broccoli.

PRAWN AND VEGETABLE STIR-FRY

Serves 4

1 tablespoon olive oil
110g (4oz) onions, chopped
110g (4oz) broccoli, divided into florets
110g (4oz) carrots, cut into small matchstick-sized pieces
110g (4oz) leeks, thinly sliced
225g (8oz) peeled prawns
50g (2oz) courgettes, thinly sliced
110g (4oz) Chinese leaves, roughly chopped
1 tablespoon grated ginger
1 small packet beansprouts
1 apple, cored and diced
1 tablespoon lemon juice

- Heat the oil in a wok or large frying pan.
- Fry the onion until soft.
- Add the broccoli, carrots and leeks and cook for 3 minutes.
- Add the prawns, courgettes, Chinese leaves, ginger, beansprouts, apple and lemon juice and cook for a further 2 minutes. Serve with salad.

VEGETABLE AND FISH KEBABS

Serves 4

450g (1lb) fish such as monkfish, red mullet, scallops, baby squid, large raw prawns
225g (8oz) cherry tomatoes
150g (5½oz) button mushrooms
1 red pepper, deseeded and cut into cubes
1 green pepper, deseeded and cut into cubes
3 small courgettes cut into 2.5cm (1in) chunks
30ml (1fl oz) olive oil
30ml (1fl oz) lemon juice
2 tablespoons chopped fresh basil
ground black pepper

- Cut the fish into bite-sized pieces.
- Thread the fish, tomatoes and vegetables on to skewers, alternating them.
- Mix together the oil, lemon juice, basil and black pepper.
- Meanwhile, heat the barbecue or grill up to temperature, pour the marinade over the raw kebabs, and cook until ready – approximately 10 minutes. Serve with salad or steamed or roasted vegetables.

Note: for best results, partially cook the peppers and courgettes by blanching in boiling water for a couple of minutes, drain and cool.

FISH AND LEEK CRUMBLE

Serves 4

4 medium leeks
2 pieces white fish of your choice
850ml ($1^1/_2$ pints) water
a small handful of peppercorns
2 teaspoons dried marjoram
3 tablespoons arrowroot
150ml (5fl oz) soya milk
salt to taste

for the crumble topping
225g (8oz) millet flakes
75g (3oz) nuts (hazelnuts, cashews or almonds)
salt
50g (2oz) organic butter

- Preheat the oven to 180°C/350°F/gas mark 4.
- Trim and chop the leeks coarsely. Put the fish and leeks in a heavy pan with the water, peppercorns and the marjoram.
- Bring to the boil and simmer for 10–15 minutes or until the fish is cooked.
- Remove the fish from the pan and leave to cool.
- Mix the arrowroot with the soya milk and add it to the cooking liquid. Mix well and continue to simmer until the liquid thickens.
- Season to taste with the salt. Put the fish into a baking dish and pour over the leeks and juices.
- To make the crumble, process the millet flakes for a couple of minutes. Mix with the nuts, salt and the organic butter.
- Spread over the fish and leek mixture and cook for 30 minutes or until lightly browned. Serve with salad or steamed vegetables.

KEDGEREE

Serves 4

175g (6oz) haddock (not smoked), filleted and skinned
75g (3oz) brown rice
30ml (1fl oz) organic, live, plain yogurt
1/2 green pepper, deseeded and chopped
1 onion, finely chopped
sprig of parsley, chopped
freshly ground black pepper
2 slices lemon to garnish

- Cover the fish with water in a shallow pan. Heat gently and poach for about 8–10 minutes. Remove the fish and flake.
- Boil the rice in the poaching water left in the pan according to the instructions on the packet. You may need to add extra water. Drain the rice, stir in the fish, yogurt, green pepper, onion and parsley and mix well.
- Heat gently, stirring all the time.
- Season with pepper, and serve garnished with lemon.

Note: as it contains rice, this kedgeree is best for lunch rather than your evening meal.

SEEDED TOFU PATTIES

Serves 4

175g (6oz) leeks
110g (4oz) carrots
110g (4oz) mushrooms
1 teaspoon olive oil
1 teaspoon oregano
50g (2oz) buckwheat or millet flakes
225g (8oz) tofu, thoroughly mashed
30ml (1fl oz) tahini
30ml (1fl oz) tamari
salt and pepper to taste
40g ($1^1/_2$ oz) sesame seeds

- Chop the leeks finely, coarsely grate the carrots and slice the mushrooms. Put the oil into a heavy-based pan and heat. Add the prepared vegetables and sauté for about 8 minutes.
- Remove from the heat, add the oregano, buckwheat or millet flakes, tofu, tahini, tamari and season with salt and pepper. Stir the mixture well and then leave to cool for a few minutes.
- Divide the mixture into 8 portions and mould each one into a ball. Roll each ball in sesame seeds until well covered, then flatten into burger shapes.
- Grill or fry for about 5 minutes on each side. Serve with salad or steamed seasonal vegetables.

SNACKS

Eating small, nutritious snacks mid-morning and mid-afternoon, between meals, will help to stabilise your blood sugar levels. Always include a protein with your snacks if you can.

An apple with four almonds

Raw celery, carrot or broccoli dipped in hummus

145g (5oz) pot organic, plain, live yogurt (with seeds or fresh fruit – optional)

Fresh fruit with 1/2 tablespoon pumpkin or sunflower seeds

1/2 avocado eaten with a teaspoon – add hummus if you like

Crudités (chopped raw vegetables) with a tofu or tahini dip

To make the tofu dip blend together:

75g (3oz) tofu
1/2 ripe avocado
1/2 garlic clove, peeled and crushed
2 spring onions, trimmed and finely chopped
2 tablespoons chopped parsley
1 teaspoon tamari sauce
75ml (3fl oz) soya, oat or rice milk (or as much as you need to achieve the desired consistency)
black pepper to taste

1 oatcake spread with mackerel pâté, sunflower seed spread, nut butters, tahini or hummus

To make the mackerel pâté blend together:

50g (2oz) smoked mackerel fillets
75g (3oz) organic, live, plain yogurt
1 tablespoon lemon juice
grated lemon rind
black pepper to taste

Handful of nuts and raisins (make sure that you have more nuts than raisins)

Carrot and cucumber sticks with hummus (not low-fat hummus as the 'fat' in hummus is an essential fatty acid which comes from tahini (sesame paste); it is good for you so you don't want it removed)

Celery sticks filled with peanut butter

Small bowl of organic, live, plain yogurt on its own or with berries

Oatcakes or rye cracker with hummus or taramasalata (not the bright pink version; get one that says 'natural' – it is quite pale pink)

Handful of nuts and seeds: make your own tasty mix by buying big bags of pumpkin, sunflower, pine kernels, linseeds and sesame seeds, putting equal quantities of each on to a baking tray and toasting them lightly in a medium oven until lightly brown. Sprinkle with tamari (wheat-free soya sauce), allow to cool, then store in an airtight container.

• HOW TO EAT OUT •

Italian: avoid pasta and pizza – choose fish, vegetables, salads, avocados and mozzarella.

Indian: avoid rice and naan bread – choose prawn, vegetable and bean (like chick pea) dishes.

Chinese: avoid rice and noodles – choose fish, egg and vegetable dishes.

Thai: avoid rice and noodles – choose fish dishes, vegetables and look for tofu curries.

Always ask to have the carbohydrate part of your meal replaced with extra vegetables or salad, and always avoid the bread tray at the beginning of the meal. If you're eating late in the evening, make sure that you have had an additional snack (when dinner should have been) so that your low blood sugar levels don't draw you to inappropriate choices.

If you are eating in somebody else's home ask for more vegetables and salad to have with the protein part of the meal and either avoid or just have a small serving of potatoes or rice.

DESSERTS

For the first three months, try to avoid having fruit after the evening meal as it is high in fructose and it is better to avoid this just before going to bed. If you would like a dessert after lunch, especially at weekends, try having a plain, organic, live yogurt and add some berries or other fruit. You could also bake an eating apple (don't use cooking apples as they are too tart) – take out the core and stuff with nuts, sultanas and cinnamon. Alternatively, try making buckwheat pancakes stuffed with a berry mix (use buckwheat flour – buckwheat is actually a vegetable not a grain – an egg and non-dairy milk).

MOVING ON

Once the first three months are up and you have trimmed your waist it will be safer to widen your food choices and start reintroducing carbohydrates such as brown rice into your evening meal. See Chapter 11 for maintenance suggestions, or try following the recommendations in my book *Natural Alternatives to Dieting* which explains how to keep eating healthily to maintain the weight that you want.

CASE STUDY

Let's take a look at the lifestyle of a woman who thinks she is doing the best she can, but still can't shift the fat around her middle. I will then show how simple it can be to change eating habits to achieve maximum fat loss.

• HELP, I'M FAT AROUND THE MIDDLE! •

I have dieted and exercised all my life in a pathetic attempt to be slimmer. The only time I was satisfied with my body was in my mid-twenties when I was living an extremely unhealthy life of immense stress, smoking and partying hard.

However, after three big children my torso is a disaster. My stomach muscles came apart and will not go back. They are strong, but simply can't hold together in the middle. Despite diet and exercise, after the second baby I was not able to shed the new fat on my tummy (I seem to have developed a new area of fat, high, under the bust) and it just got worse during the third pregnancy, despite an extremely healthy diet and lots of walking. I have never had a waist. Even as a teenager I wore men's jeans because I was straight up and down rather than waisted, so a nipped waist is not something I aspire to. However, I know that whenever I gain weight it goes on around my middle and in the old days when I lost weight it went from my chest and stomach.

Not any more. I'm now forty-one, had my kids in my late thirties, so I know that's partly to blame. Stress is also a huge factor. When I worked full time my job was extremely stressful, I spent nearly three years juggling motherhood with commuting and working full time and the memory of the stress still haunts me.

However, for the last five years I've been working from home as a freelancer and am extremely unstressed. Yes, I've got three kids as challenging as any, and I do work part time, but I wouldn't want things any different, and I do sleep well.

I have stuck to a very healthy diet high in fruit and vegetables and whole foods for more than two years. I have always exercised, either running or gym or mountain biking.

On good days I eat like a monk but my downfall is picking off the children's plates (I can't stand waste) and nibbling at home in the evenings. I've recently tried avoiding sugar altogether and it seems to be helping with my evening snacking.

I suspect I may have some form of insulin resistance (I've noticed if I do have sugar I can have crashing energy lows a few hours later, when I think I must be coming down with flu or something), and I may have some form of intolerance to wheat (bloating) and dairy (fantastic burps).

So that's the story. Now, below are examples of this woman's typical eating regime, followed in each case by my suggestions for simple changes that could really help her body to let go of its fat-around-the-middle pattern.

Day 1

What she ate and drank

7.00	Get up
7.30	Cup of tea with milk
8.00	Cornflakes with milk and a teaspoon of sugar sprinkled on the top
11.00	Latte
12.30	Cheese baguette
3.00	Bag of nuts and raisins
4.00	Latte
6.00	Apple
8.00	Cauliflower cheese, French beans, 1 glass wine, 2 peaches
10.00	Cup of redbush (Rooibos) tea with milk
11.00	Bed

What she did wrong

The first problem with the food and drink on Day 1 is that the day starts with a shot of caffeine and milk (containing lactose – milk sugar), after what is effectively a fast from the evening meal the night before. So straight away the body is stimulated and up goes the blood sugar and then out comes the cortisol. This woman has set herself up to fail from the beginning of the day. The message her body has got is to store food as fat, not burn it as energy. Half an hour later comes a large helping of sugar both from the cornflakes, which can anyway contain quite a bit of sugar in different guises e.g. sucrose, glucose, plus the extra teaspoon. The cheese baguette at lunchtime is too much carbohydrate compared to the protein from the cheese and the baguette is white refined flour and so will be digested quickly causing a rise in insulin. This woman is not eating an enormous amount of food or pigging out on chocolate but her body is storing every bit it can.

Alternative 'lose-your-belly' day 1

7.00	Get up
7.30	Cup of hot water with slice of lemon (acts as a detox to the liver) or peppermint or redbush tea (leave out the milk or use soya, rice or oat milk over the next three months)
8.00	Sugar-free muesli (boosted with seeds) with organic soya milk, rice or oat milk and a cup of redbush, peppermint or camomile tea

11.00	Grain coffee made with frothy, heated organic soya milk and an apple
1.00	Either tuna salad open sandwich on rye bread or, even better, salad (with quinoa) and hummus
4.00	Grain coffee or herb tea, handful of nuts
6.00	Apple
8.00	Cauliflower cheese, French beans, 1 glass wine, 2 peaches
10.00	Cup of redbush tea without milk
11.00	Bed

Day 2

What she ate and drank

7.30	Get up
8.00	Two cups of tea with milk
8.30	Commercial breakfast cereal with milk
12.00	Cup of coffee
1.00	Carrot, tomato, red pepper with hummus and a slice of wholemeal toast (with extra seeds)
2.00	Cup of tea and satsuma
4.00	Chocolate bar
5.00	Cup of tea
5.30	Meat balls, white rice, vegetable purée sauce
8.00	Three glasses of wine and packet of crisps, handful of prunes
11.00	Bed

What she did wrong

Again she starts the day off by giving the wrong message to her body, but this time the effect is stronger as there are two cups of tea. The other problem is the virtual four-hour fast from one o'clock to five thirty broken only by caffeine (from the tea and chocolate), sugar and one satsuma. You should never go for more than three hours without proper food. This woman's body thinks it is under attack because the gaps without 'proper' food along with the stimulant effects of the food and drink she has had will cause the release of the stress hormones. Unfortunately, the three glasses of wine, potato crisps and dried fruit (prunes) are not a good mix in terms of blood sugar and a lethal combination in the evening before going to bed because together they raise blood sugar, increase insulin and, as the digestion slows overnight, encourage the body to store more fat. It is made even worse because there is no protein (animal or vegetable) to slow this fat-building effect.

Alternative 'lose-your-belly' day 2

7.30 Get up
8.00 Cup of hot water with lemon and one cup of redbush or peppermint tea with soya, rice or oat milk
8.30 Sugar-free muesli with soya milk
11.00 Grain coffee and apple
1.00 Carrot, tomato, red pepper with hummus and a slice of rye toast (with extra seeds)
2.00 Redbush tea and satsuma
4.00 Bag of nuts and raisins or oatcake with nut butter
5.00 Cup of redbush tea
5.30 Piece of fish, no rice (just for the first three months, then use brown rice), vegetable purée sauce (sugar free) and vegetables like broccoli, carrots
8.00 Stick to one glass of wine at weekends only for the first three months, fresh fruit salad, with nuts and seeds and a live, plain, organic yogurt or a bowl of soup (either tinned or instant miso soup for speed)
11.00 Bed

Day 3

What she ate and drank

7.00 Get up
7.30 Cup of tea
8.00 White toast with margarine
9.30 Cup of tea
10.30 Cup of tea
11.30 Cup of tea
12.00 Chicken, courgette in spicy beans with broccoli
1.00 Two satsumas
1.30 Cup of coffee
5.00 Glass of squash
5.30 Very small plate of spaghetti bolognaise (rejected by the kids), six chips
6.00 Pear
9.00 A corn on the cob (bit of olive oil), two thirds of a box of strawberries, twenty small organic wheat crackers
10.00 Cup of redbush tea
11.00 Bed

What she did wrong

Well, the day starts the same – a twelve-hour fast followed by a shot of caffeine. Then white refined carbohydrate toast and trans fats from the margarine. After the toast there is a four-hour gap (one hour too long) punctuated with three shots of caffeine from three cups of tea. Her body is starting to think the famine is back and triggers a stress response which is compounded by the stress hormones triggered by the tea. The stress of rushing around after the children will be adding to this. The shot of sugar in the glass of squash is not a healthy choice. The meal at five thirty is small but contains a lot of starchy carbohydrate from the white spaghetti and the chips. When she does sit down to eat properly at nine the food she chooses does not contain any protein, needed to keep the blood sugar stable. This is probably why she could not control her consumption of crackers.

Alternative 'lose-your-belly' day 3

7.00	Get up
7.30	Cup of hot water and lemon
8.00	Porridge oats made with water and sprinkled with nuts and berries or a piece of rye toast with organic butter
9.30	Cup of redbush tea
10.30	Cup of peppermint tea with some nuts
12.00	Chicken (or fish would be better), courgette in spicy beans with broccoli
1.00	Two satsumas
1.30	Cup of grain coffee
5.00	Glass of diluted pure orange juice with an oatcake and hummus (protein from the chick peas in the hummus)
5.30	Small plate of corn pasta with spaghetti sauce and tuna
6.00	Pear with a handful of nuts
9.00	A corn on the cob (bit of olive oil), slices of pan-fried tofu sprinkled with tamari soya sauce (takes five minutes) or quick scrambled egg, small salad
10.00	Redbush tea
11.00	Bed

• 'LOSE-YOUR-BELLY' MEAL COMPARISON •

You can have your own personal meal comparison to show how what you are eating now compares to what you should be eating. See Resources, page 183 or go directly to www.naturalhealthpractice.com/fataroundthemiddle to find out how you can get your own tailor-made programme.

CHEAT DAYS

As I said earlier, this three-month 'lose-your-belly' plan will work effectively as long as you stick to it 80 per cent of the time. But because we are all only human, I've tried to make it easier still by offering you 'cheat days' during which you can eat and drink whatever and however much you want.

- At the end of the first month – have one cheat day
- During the second month – have one cheat day a fortnight
- During the third month – have one cheat day a week

By giving yourself permission to cheat, you will remove any guilt attached to 'going off the rails'. You may also find that you don't cheat anywhere near as much as you think you're going to. There's nothing like being told we can't have something to make us want it even more. So once you are told that you can eat whatever you want, you will find that you do not go very mad at all.

SUPPLEMENTS

Supplementation is an integral part of the programme. I feel very strongly that the correct combination of supplements (see Chapter 5) will enhance and improve all the good things you are doing with your new eating plan, making your dietary changes much more effective.

You will only be following this intensive programme for a period of three months, after which you can cut back to a maintenance programme to keep things ticking over. It may cost a bit to turn your health around, but for the price of a haircut you are not only going to look and feel good, but also increase your chances of good health in the future.

Choosing supplements

Walk into any chemist, supermarket or health-food shop and you will be faced with a huge selection of supplements. It can be utterly baffling to know which brand to choose. When it comes to buying supplements, my view is that you get what you pay for. I always advise clients to buy the highest quality (which usually means the most expensive) that they can afford. In particular I recommend BioCare, Solgar and The Natural Health Practice.

You need to get good-quality supplements for maximum absorption. Capsules (if possible vegetable ones instead of gelatine) are preferable to tablets as they tend to be filled only with the essential nutrients, whereas tablets can include a variety of fillers, binders and bulking agents.

Mineral supplements like calcium should be in the form of citrates, ascorbates or polynicotinates, which are more easily absorbed by the body. Chlorides, sulphates, carbonates and oxides should be avoided as they are not so easily assimilated and mineral supplements in this form may pass through the body without being absorbed.

When choosing amino acids, look out for the difference between two different forms: L- or D-, for example L-arginine or D-arginine. The L- forms are those that are found in Nature, whereas the D- forms are synthetic. So opt for the L- forms as these are closest to those found in food. Amino acids should always be taken on an empty stomach.

Your supplement programme

The aim is to control high levels of stress hormones by getting your blood sugar in balance and looking at the stress in your life. Supplements will enable your body to do this more efficiently and within our three-month time frame.

You need the following daily:

Chromium	200mcg	Siberian ginseng	100mg
Zinc	15mg	Co-enzyme Q10	25mg
Vitamin E (mixed tocopherols)	300ius	Alpha lipoic acid	100mg
Manganese	5mg	Green tea extract	50mg
Magnesium	300mg		
Vitamin B1	25mg	*Amino acids*	
Vitamin B2	25mg	N-acetyl cysteine	500mg
Vitamin B3	25mg	L-carnitine	200mg
Vitamin B12	25mcg	L-tyrosine	200mg
Biotin	35mcg	L-arginine	200mg
Folic acid	200mcg	L-glutamine	200mg
Vitamin B5	50mg	Isoleucine	100mg
Vitamin B6		Leucine	100mg
(as pyridoxal-5-phosphate)	25mg	Valine	100mg

It can seem terribly confusing when you see a long list of supplements that you need to take, and it can be quite daunting trying to make sure that you are getting the right ones. To make it easier for you I have asked The Natural Health Practice to help formulate two special supplements. The first, 'Lose your Belly' Nutri Plus contains all the vitamins, minerals and other nutrients mentioned above, in the right amounts; the second, 'Lose your Belly' Amino Plus contains all the amino acids mentioned above, in the correct amounts. They are available from www.naturalhealthpractice.com or all good health-food shops.

Along with the Nutri and the Amino, you should also take:

Vitamin C (as ascorbate) with bioflavonoids	1,000mg
Omega 3 fish oil	1,000mg

And if your stress levels are extremely high then I would suggest adding:

Rhodiola rosea	250mg

EXERCISE

The most effective approach to exercise in terms of losing that fat around your middle is a two-pronged attack comprising aerobic and weight-training exercises. This will give you the best results in the fastest time.

Note: if you have not exercised for some time, do check with your doctor before embarking on an exercise programme.

The best way to do aerobic exercise

Aim for four thirty-minute sessions of continuous aerobic exercise each week and choose something that you enjoy so that you are more than likely to stick with it. This can include fast walking, dancing, swimming, jogging or an exercise class. The aim is to feel slightly out of breath but not so much that you cannot carry on a conversation. If you can speak whilst exercising it means that you are still getting a good supply of oxygen and a greater proportion of fat will be burned.

To get the absolute best out of your aerobic exercise you should vary its intensity with what the experts call 'interval training'. If you are out for a brisk walk, for instance, pick a point between two trees or two lampposts, and walk really fast (or break into a jog) just for that distance, dropping back into your slower pace to recover afterwards. Repeat this, pushing yourself just a little bit harder each time. If you are on a treadmill, either choose the interval training programme, which varies the intensity of your workout, or adapt the speed and inclination so that you are periodically puffed out. Then return to normal once more so that you can recover before going faster again.

For example, depending on your level of fitness when starting, if you were on the treadmill you could:

- start walking at 6kph or any level you are comfortable with
- after one minute increase the speed to 6.5
- after the next minute increase to 7.0
- after the next minute increase to 7.5
- after the next minute increase to 8.0
- after the next minute increase to 8.5
- after the next minute (so that you have done five minutes in total), go back to 6
- after the next minute step up the pace to 6.5 again, and so on.

You should aim to keep this up for twenty to thirty minutes.

By varying the speeds and gaps as you get fitter you will keep your body 'on its toes', so that it stays in fat-burning mode. This can also help to make a simple walk on the treadmill a bit more of a challenge and more interesting too.

The best way to do weights

In addition to your four thirty-minute sessions of aerobic activity each week, you should try to do two or three thirty-minute sessions of weight-/resistance-training. It sounds like a lot, but you could easily combine thirty minutes of each type of exercise in a one-hour session. If you can manage that three times during the week, you will only have to fit in a thirty-minute walk at some time over the weekend.

After weight-training it is important to give your muscles the chance to recover and repair themselves, so it's not a good idea to train the same muscle groups every day. Your body builds muscle when you are resting (remember, this burns fat!), so if you've worked really hard on one part of your body, allow that part to rest for at least four days. The best advice is to concentrate on your upper body in one session, then on your lower body in the next, so that each muscle group has time to recover.

Always tackle the weight-training part of your workout before the aerobics to ensure that you do not exhaust your muscles and that you have the strength to weight-train properly. The best time to exercise is early in the morning as this is when the body is most inclined to burn stored fat. Try to have some sort of protein (nuts or a tuna salad) within half an hour of exercise (whether aerobic or weight-training). The protein feeds the muscles used during the training and helps to restore them.

Weight-training at home

There are lots of really good exercise videos on the market (but make sure that you get one made by a fitness expert rather than a celebrity). These may encourage you to work with weighted dumbbells or stretchy rubber bands, which are inexpensive and can be bought at most sports shops.

I have listed some resistance exercises below to get you started at home using a litre bottle of water or bags of rice (brown of course, only joking!) as weights.

When you work with weights the technique is really important; if you are not getting it right you will either be wasting your time and effort or you could end up injuring yourself. It can be helpful to perform the exercises in front of a mirror to make sure that you are doing them correctly.

When using weights for the first time, always start with a light weight and build up slowly. The aim is to lift the weight twelve times (this is called a repetition or rep) and do three lots of these (called sets). You will know that you have the right weight (for now) if you find it quite difficult to finish the third set and maybe only get to about eight or ten. If you can do more than twelve reps the weight is too light. Allow yourself around one minute to rest between sets. You will find that you gain strength quickly, so as soon as the third set becomes easier, increase either the weight or the resistance.

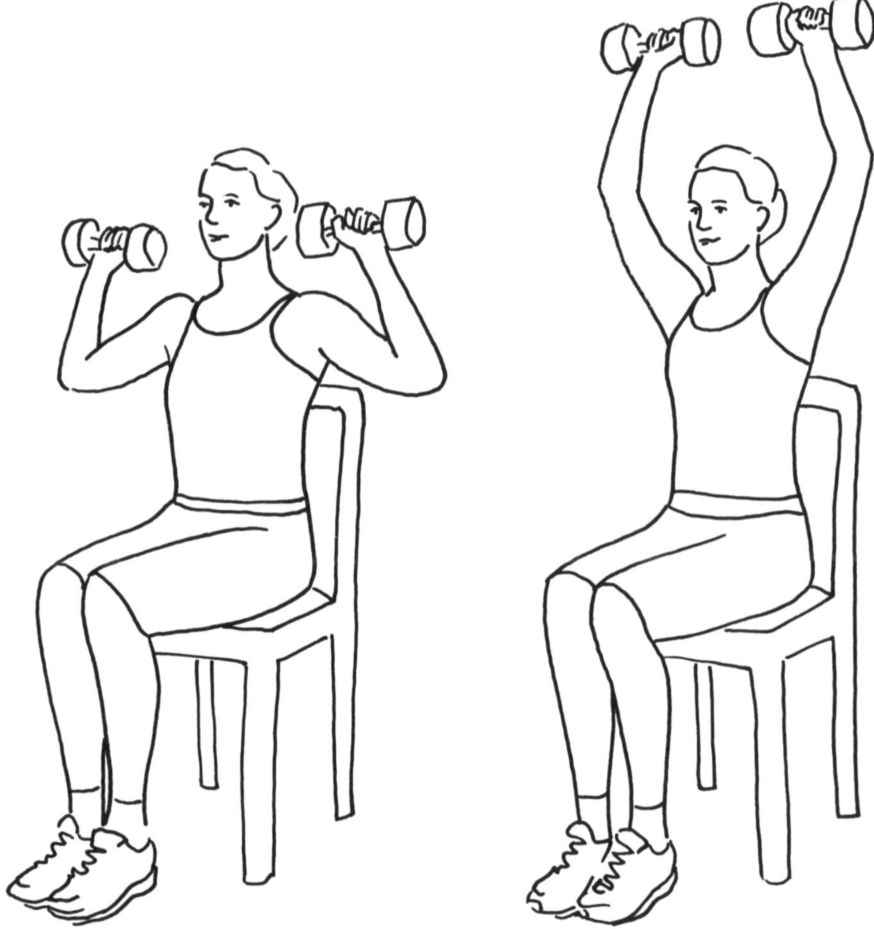

SEATED OVERHEAD PRESS

What it works: arms and shoulders.

1. Sit on a stool or at the end of a bench with your feet flat on the floor. Hold a weight in each hand so that it is level with your ears. Your palms should be facing forwards, with your elbows out.

2. Press the weights upwards and inwards in a smooth movement until they nearly touch above your head. Your arms should now be almost straight, with your elbows just short of locked. Slowly lower the weights back to the starting position.

Safety tip: Do not lean backwards – stay upright with your chin up, shoulders squared and chest high.

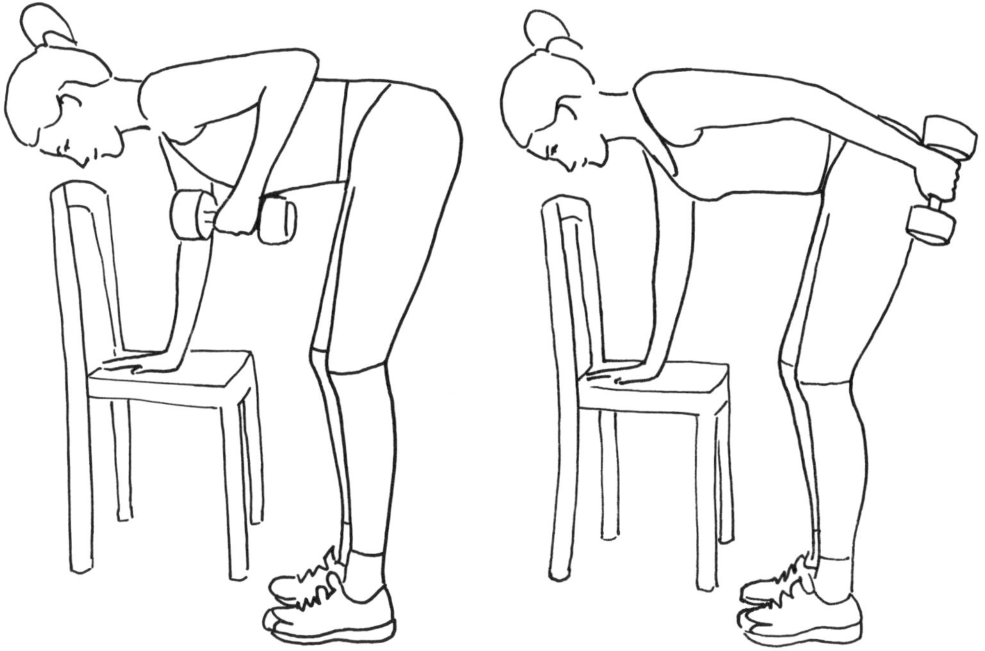

TRICEPS KICKBACK

What it works: back of upper arms.

1. Stand at arm's distance from a bench with your feet hip-width apart. Rest your right palm on the surface of the bench and bend your knees slightly so your back is parallel to the floor. Start with your left elbow pulled up, your upper arm parallel to the floor.

2. Keeping your upper arm still, straighten your left arm, bringing the weight back and up to your hip, until your arm is fully extended and parallel to the floor (without locking your elbow). Hold; then slowly bend the arm back to the starting position. Complete your reps; then switch sides.

Safety tip: Make sure your back remains level, and parallel to the floor. Do not lift one shoulder higher than the other.

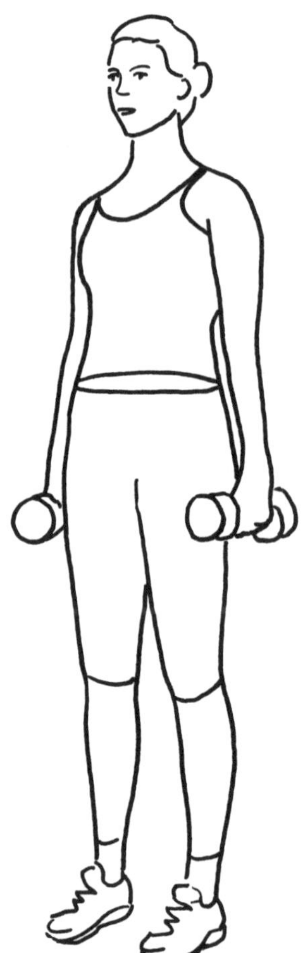

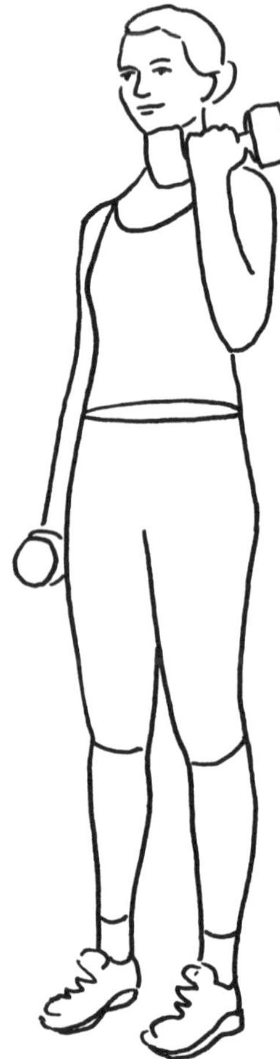

ALTERNATING BICEP CURL

What it works: arms and shoulders.

1. Stand with your legs straight but not locked, feet hip-width apart. Hold a weight in each hand, arms by your sides, palms facing inwards.

2. Keeping your upper arm still, bend your left elbow and raise the weight up and in towards your shoulder. As it reaches your shoulder, rotate your palm so that it faces inwards. Hold; then slowly lower. Repeat with the right arm and keep alternating sides for the set.

Safety tip: Don't arch your back – keep it straight and still at all times. Keep your elbows tucked into your side throughout the exercise; don't allow them to move in front of your body.

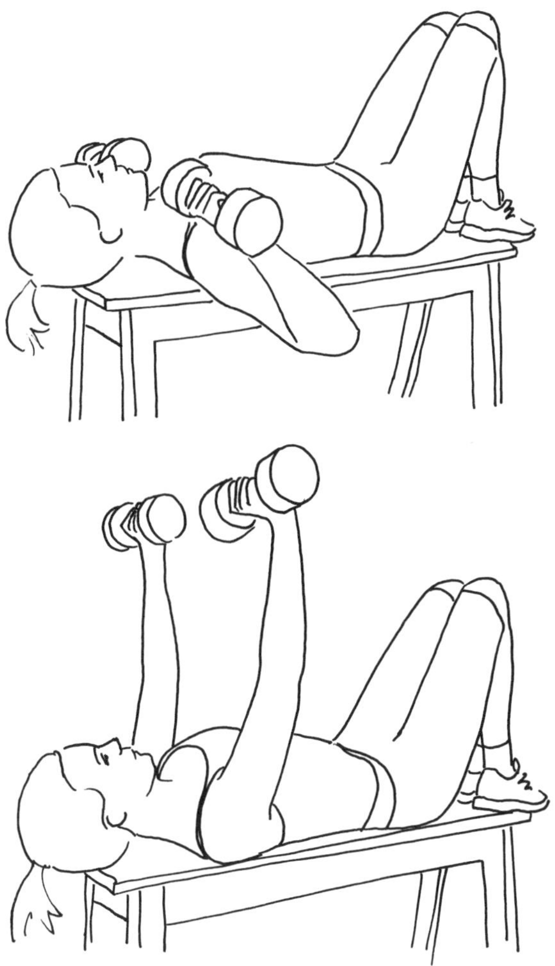

Bench Press

What it works: chest, shoulders and the back of the arms.

1. Lie on your back on a bench with your knees bent. Hold a weight in each hand at chest level, with your palms facing towards your feet and elbows out.

2. Press the weights straight up, without locking the elbow joints, until they're right over your collarbone. Then slowly lower them to the starting position, feeling the stretch in your chest muscles as your elbows drop below the level of the bench.

Safety tip: Keep your head rested on the bench at all times. Don't let the weights sway back towards your head and over your face; lift them in one smooth movement.

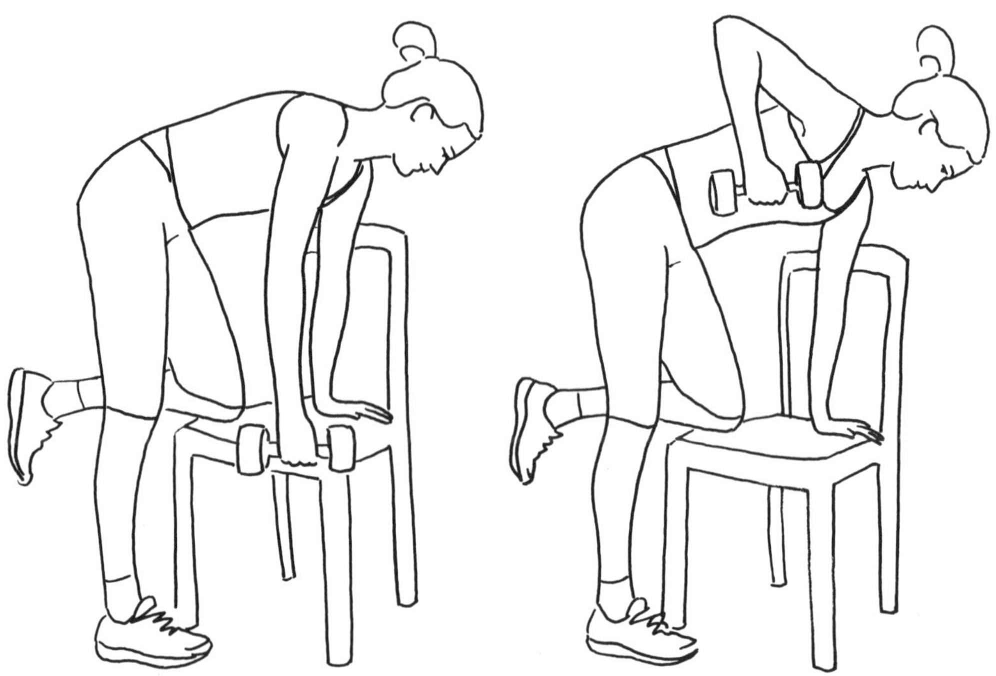

SINGLE-ARM ROW

What it works: back.

1. Start with your right foot flat on the floor and your left knee resting on a flat bench. Lean forwards and rest your left arm on the bench; your back should be almost parallel with the floor. Take a weight in your right hand, with your arm hanging straight down, palm turned in towards your body and your thumb facing forwards.

2. Pull your elbow up to bring the weight roughly parallel with your torso. Hold; then slowly lower it to the starting position. After you complete the planned number of reps for your right arm, follow the same instructions for your left.

Safety tip: Don't move anything other than the working arm. Keep your back flat and avoid rounding or hunching it.

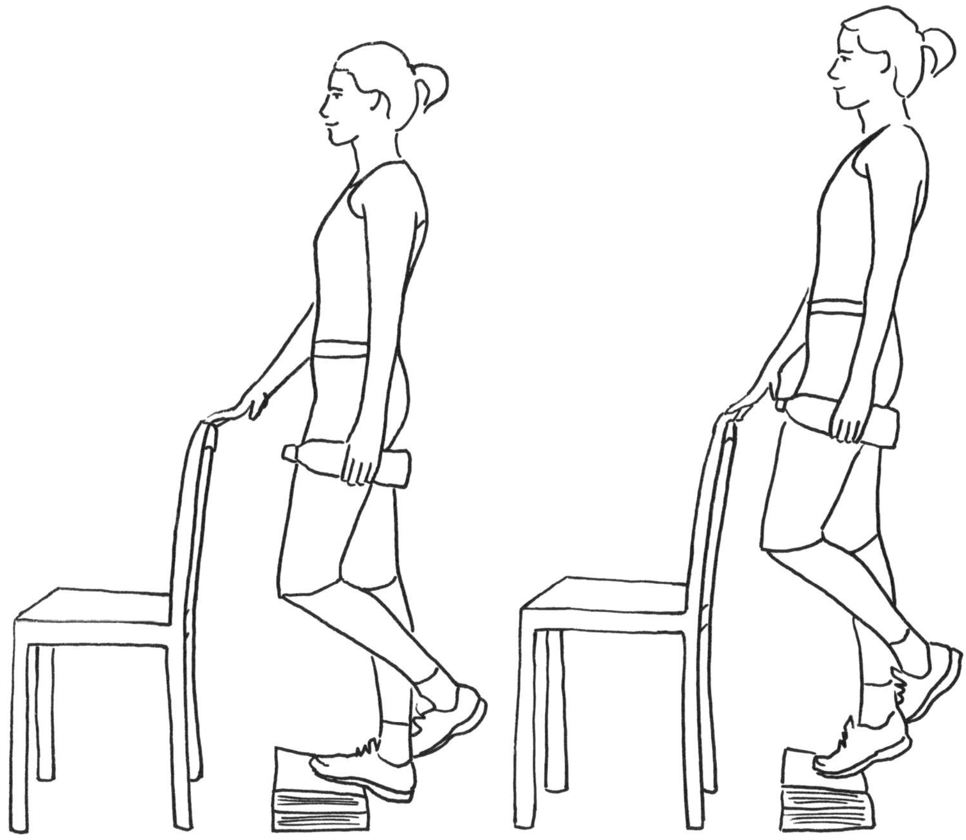

Single-leg Calf Raise

What it works: calf muscles.

1. Hold on to a chair for balance with your right hand, and hold a weight in your left hand, palm facing in. Stand on the ball of your right foot on a step or a couple of big books. Lift your left foot and hook it behind your right calf. Lower your right heel as far as you can, feeling the stretch on your calf at the bottom.

2. Using your calf muscle, raise yourself up on to the toes of your right foot. Pause in that position, then slowly lower back to the starting position. Repeat for the planned number of reps. Switch legs and hands and follow the same instructions on the other side.

Safety tip: Put your weight squarely on the ball of your foot. Don't lean forwards; maintain an upright posture.

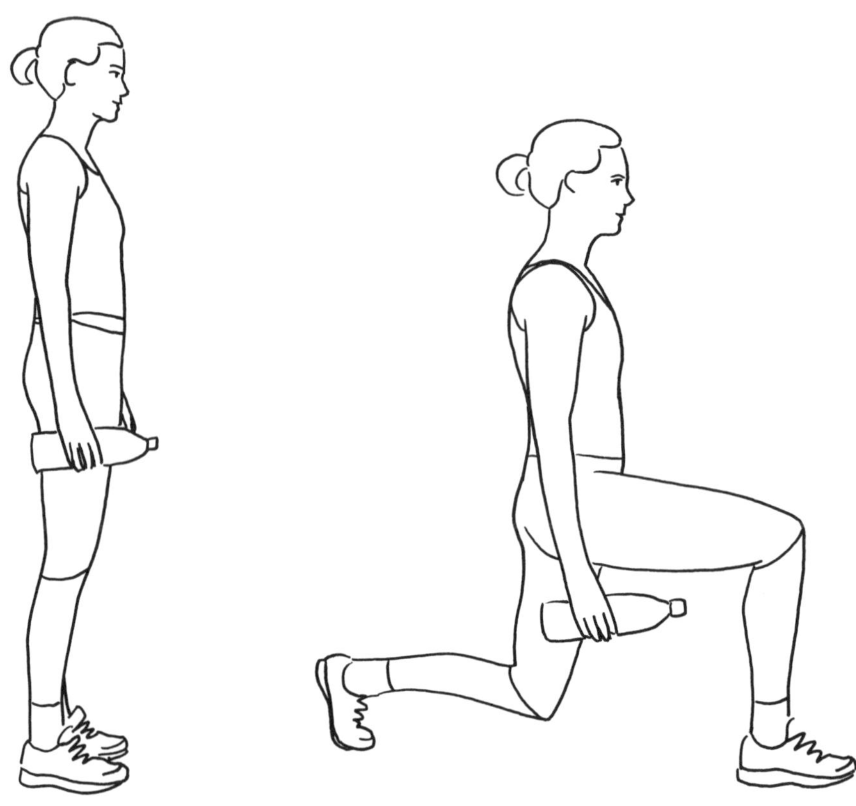

ALTERNATING LUNGES

What it works: legs.

1. Stand with your feet shoulder-width apart and a weight in each hand.

2. Lunge forward with your right foot, bending the leg until your knee is over your foot, thigh parallel to the floor. Your left leg should be extended behind you, knee slightly bent with your left heel raised above the floor. Pause, then push with your right leg back into the starting position. Repeat with your left leg.

Safety tip: Make sure the front knee never extends beyond your foot, as this will place excessive strain on the knee joints.

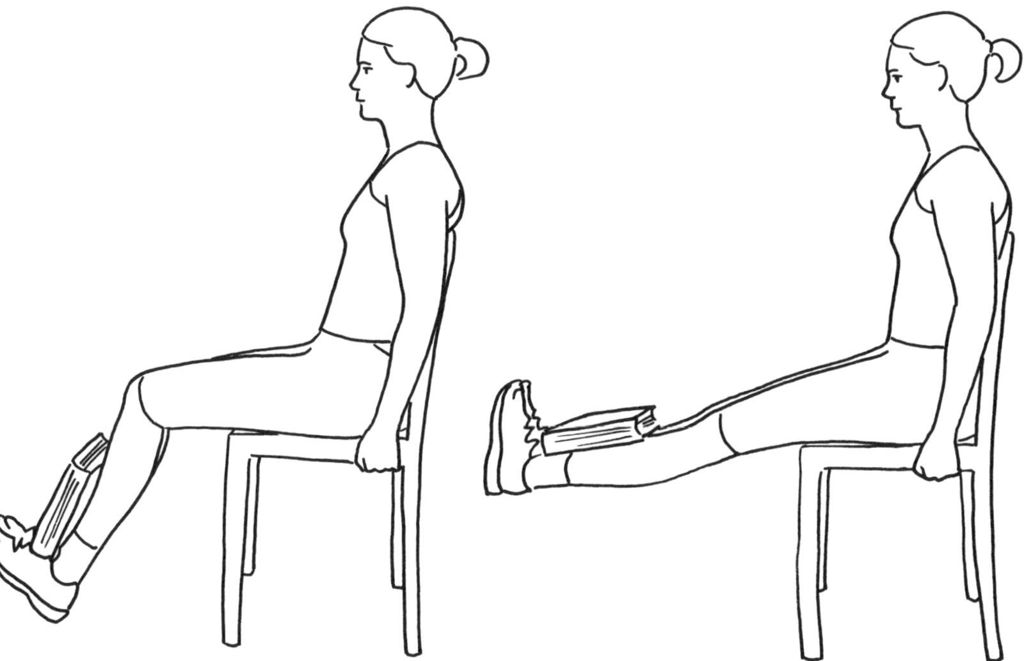

LEG EXTENSION WITH BOOK

What it works: thighs.

1. Sit on a chair or bench, legs slightly apart. Place a big book (e.g. telephone directory) on your shins and support it by pointing your toes upwards. Steady yourself by holding on to the base of the chair.

2. Raise your legs until they are straight out in front of you. Flex the quadriceps at the top of the movement, before lowering your legs back towards the floor. Don't let your heels touch the floor between reps; lower them to just above the floor to ensure continuous tension.

Safety tip: Keep your back straight at all times.

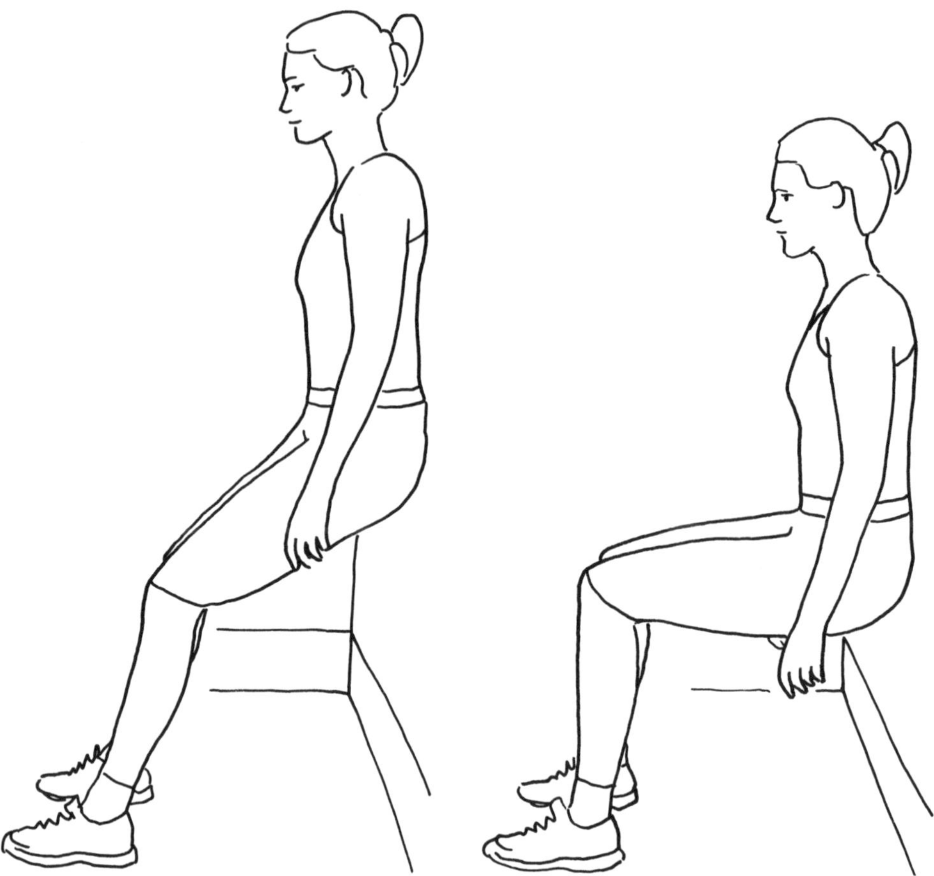

THE INVISIBLE CHAIR

What it works: thighs and buttocks.

1. Stand leaning with your back against a wall, knees slightly bent, feet a little further than shoulder-width apart.

2. Slowly lower yourself until your thighs are parallel to the floor with your knees above your feet. Hold the position for as long as possible.

Safety tip: Don't let your knees extend over your toes as this puts excessive strain on the knee joints.

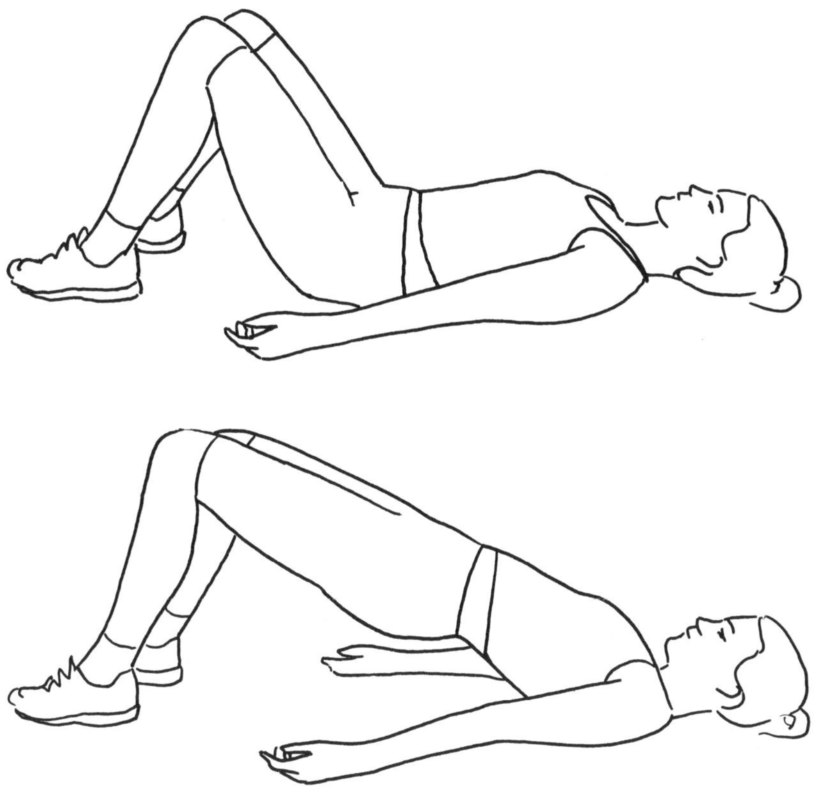

Butt Squeeze

What it works: buttocks.

1. Lie on a mat on your back with your feet shoulder-width apart and your knees bent.

2. Press through your feet to lift your buttocks off the floor, exhaling as you do so. Push your pelvis up to bring it in line with your thighs and upper body. Squeeze your buttocks for 1 second. Inhale as you slowly return to the starting position.

These exercises are designed just to get you started. There are many other exercises you can do for the same body part and also machines that can be used at the gym. The rowing and cross-training machines are also good as they work both the lower and upper body at the same time. Make sure that you are instructed properly in how to use the rowing machine as you can strain your back if your technique is not correct.

LIFESTYLE

This is the stress-busting part of your plan of action. For some it might be the easiest bit, for others the hardest. But it is as important as nutrition, supplements and exercise if you really are going to trim that waist and get healthy.

As I explained in Chapter 7, getting rid of the weight around your middle depends largely on reducing levels of the stress hormones, especially cortisol. So you need to take a long, hard look at the stress in your life to see what you can and cannot control.

Think about whether there are any fundamental changes you could make. Perhaps review your goals and expectations or manage your time more effectively? Look at my suggestions on pages 112–115 for possible adjustments you could make, as well as ideas for relaxation. Remember that getting this part of the plan right is crucial to making it work for you.

Quick relaxation technique

When time is tight and you feel wound up and in a rush, try this quick relaxation technique. It takes only one minute – and it's worth it, even if you really don't think you have one minute to spare. Just do it and watch time expand.

- Find a quiet spot and sit upright in a comfortable chair with both your feet flat on the ground.
- Close your eyes.
- Place your right hand loosely on your belly and your left hand on top of it.
- Breathe in deeply and at the same time repeat this sentence mentally to yourself, adding your name at the beginning: 'Sally, the next one minute of clock time will feel like thirty minutes of relaxation. Yes, Sally, when you have finished this relaxation, you will have received all the benefits of thirty minutes of relaxation.'
- Let out a long, slow breath and visualise the second hand of a clock slowing nearly to a stop.
- Say to yourself, 'Sally, your mind is at peace.'
- Imagine yourself in a bath of warm, soft, lovely smelling water. Feel the warm water releasing all the tension in your muscles.
- As you breathe in say, 'I can'.
- As you breathe out say, 'let go'.
- As you breathe in say, 'I am'.
- As you breathe out say, 'relaxed'.
- Visualise the clock returning to its normal speed.
- Open your eyes and have a good stretch.

KEEP IT UP

Changing the way in which you eat, adding supplements, an exercise regime and trying to cut back on the stress in your life is not going to be easy for the first few weeks. The four-point plan is a major undertaking and represents quite a significant life change. But please do persevere. There will be days when you just cannot resist that bar of chocolate or that glass of wine, when

> ### • JOINING A GYM •
>
> It might be a good idea to join a local gym if you can. The trainers there will get you started on a basic programme suited to your level and they can help you to progress as your fitness improves. Joining fees can be expensive so look out for special offers (many have recruitment drives when they slash fees once a year) and always ask for a few guest passes first so that you get a good feel for whether or not it is the right place for you. If you feel uncomfortable you will be less likely to use the gym and your money will be wasted.
>
> A local council-run gym is a good option – they are excellent value for money and usually don't require a joining fee, so you just pay as you go.
>
> If you, like many others, belong to a gym but rarely use your membership, make a concerted effort to get down there and ask for a new exercise programme. Tell the trainer what you are trying to achieve and ask them to draw up a regime that suits your fitness level and lifestyle.
>
> If you are really serious about changing your body shape you might even want to consider taking on a personal trainer, just to get you through the three-month intensive phase. They can be expensive but they can be extremely motivating and the one-on-one attention increases the chance of a positive outcome. Think of the expenditure as an investment in your long-term health and happiness, not as an indulgence. (You could also cut the cost by sharing your sessions with a friend. In fact, teaming up with someone may boost your chances of success as you can spur each other on.)

you feel the stress overwhelming you, and when it's pouring with rain and the idea of a walk is about as appealing as an enema. But keep going.

After the first few days without sugar and stimulants you might start to feel headachey and that you have a cold or the flu coming on. Your nose may start to run and your legs may ache. This is actually a good sign. Your body is starting to detoxify and it is eliminating toxins and waste products that it has been holding on to for a while. Once over those first few days you will – I promise – start to feel so much healthier than you have for a long time. A gentle jog on a sunny day can do more for your self-esteem and mood than any full-fat-milk

TIPS FOR THE EXERCISE PHOBIC

The aim is to get exercise back into your life, not to turn you into a fitness freak. If the idea of activity appals you, try thinking about it in terms of just upping a few of the small activities you do each day.

If you have not exercised for a while, start off very gently with just five to ten minutes and build it up gradually.

- Always warm up for at least five minutes before exercising.
- Always cool down after the exercise with stretching movements.
- Choose an exercise routine that fits in with your life. Dancing to music at home, for example, is fine (buy some new CDs, or a dance video).
- Why not get a rebounder (mini trampoline) or get on the kids' trampoline – it's harder work than you think.
- Get a skipping rope. Skipping is an excellent way to get the heart pumping.
- Ask your neighbours if any of them has an exercise bike/treadmill/rowing machine in their garage. So many people have them but never use them and would be only too happy to know that their expensive machinery is being put to good use.
- If you are going to exercise in the evening try to do it straight after work. There is nothing like coming home to a warm house and a beckoning television to dampen your (not-so) cast-iron willpower.
- Think about being generally more active. Walk up the stairs, instead of taking the lift or standing on the escalators. Park further away from where you need to go, or walk one stop further on before getting on the bus.
- Join a ramblers' club so that the walking becomes a social activity.
- Plan family walks/bike rides into your weekend.
- Borrow a friend's or a neighbour's dog on a regular basis. There is nothing like the pitiful look in a dog's eyes to ensure that you get out for a brisk walk/jog and they are so grateful afterwards!
- Check out classes at your local swimming pool.
- Cancel the newspaper delivery and either walk or cycle to the shop every morning. You will be saving the cost of delivery and your health.
- When you pick the kids up from school take a football along and suggest going to the park for a kickaround. Then join in – really join in and keep it all going for thirty minutes. They will be happy (if not a little amazed) and you can tick another aerobic session off your weekly list.
- Every time you plan a trip in the car stop and think. If you left a little earlier couldn't you walk there? Or cycle? Exercise is always so much more satisfying if you are killing two birds with one stone.
- Take a proper lunch break at work: go for a half-hour walk then come back and eat your lunch calmly.

full-caffeine latte can. And in less than a month you will start to notice a few changes. The fat at the top of your belly often goes first, then the fat lower down, then across your back. Before you know it, your clothes will start to feel loose and friends will be commenting on how good you look.

At certain points over the three months you might feel that you come to a full stop, and that although initially you saw a difference in your body shape, nothing now seems to be happening. Again, you should persevere, as changes will start to happen again. What you are doing is working, although you may not see it all the time. Your body has got the message to lose that belly, so stick with it. And if you need just a little extra encouragement to spur you on, get yourself a 'slimmer you' photograph (see Resources, page 183 or go directly to www.naturalhealthpractice.com/fataroundthemiddle). A photograph of you as you will look when you have shed that fat around the middle will be fantastic motivation.

This is, after all, only a three-month programme. It is not a life sentence as dieting might be (or might already have been) and I am willing to bet that once you reach your goal, you will want to keep up with a few of the changes. Scientists say it takes ten days to break a habit. So after three months some of these changes will be so much a part of your life you'll want to stay with them for ever.

Remember to record your measurements as you go along and reward yourself handsomely when you reach the end of your three months. And just to ensure that you don't duck straight back into old, bad habits take a look at the next chapter for a few tips on keeping on the straight and narrow.

• Chapter 11 •

STAYING SLIM AND HEALTHY

Once it's off, how to keep it off

Congratulations! You have achieved your goal and lost that fat around the middle. Now read on to find out how to make sure that it stays off and never returns.

FOOD AND DRINK

My advice is to resist any urge to go back to sugar and refined carbohydrates. Stick, if you can, to the 80 per cent rule (see page 135) and only indulge 20 per cent of the time. The occasional birthday cake or dessert at a special event is fine but don't let these things slip back into your everyday diet.

It is safe now to reintroduce starchy carbohydrates with your evening meal, so include brown rice, potatoes or pasta if you like. Just make sure that you still have a protein (animal or vegetable) with that meal to provide a good balance. The two foods that I would suggest you avoid most of the time (80 per cent) are sugar (in any form) and refined carbohydrates.

The sweetness in your diet over the last three months has been coming from fruit and vegetables – vegetables like parsnips and carrots can taste very sweet. A woman I saw in the clinic said that after she had eliminated sugar from her diet, then went to a party and had a piece of chocolate cake, found the sugary sweetness was overwhelming. Her taste buds had adapted to the sweetness naturally contained in fruits and vegetables.

If you do want to add more sweetness into your diet the best natural sweeteners are real maple syrup (not maple-flavoured syrup) and barley malt syrup. You can also now add in grapes, dried fruits and bananas. Bananas and dates can be used in cakes and desserts to give sweetness as well as drizzling maple syrup on your porridge in the mornings. Add some nuts or seeds to it for a shot of protein. You can make delicious sugar-free desserts – all the cakes and puddings in my book *Healthy Eating for the Menopause* are made without sugar. You would probably enjoy all the other recipes in that book for soups, main courses and snacks.

The odd cup of coffee or black tea is fine now, but judge how you feel when you drink it. If the coffee makes you feel as if you are climbing the walls then it's clear that your body cannot cope with it and you would be better off with tea or you may prefer to stick to herbal teas. Try introducing green tea if you like – it does contain caffeine but it also brings good levels of antioxidants into your diet.

Aim to continue with the pattern of eating little and often, taking healthy snacks between meals. This will keep your metabolism up and your weight down.

Widen your diet to include wheat as wholemeal bread or wholewheat pasta. But if you feel bloated or get flatulence when you add it back in, you are probably better off without it. Try spelt bread or pasta instead and see how you get on with that.

When you eat out at a restaurant, it is now fine to have the white rice or noodles. It is best to still make sure you have protein (fish or beans, for example) with the meal and to keep the white carbohydrate portion smaller than you might have done in the past. Load up your plate with salad or vegetables.

If you want to, you could now drink alcohol two or three times a week. We all need at least three alcohol-free days a week to give the liver a rest. Generally avoid beer and go for wine or spirits and limit yourself to two drinks at a time for your own general health.

Keep in your cheat day once a week. On the cheat day, eat and drink whatever and however much you want. You will find that it is much easier to stick to healthier eating for most of the week when you know there is going to be one day when you can eat whatever you want.

SUPPLEMENTS

When you have achieved the shape you want, you can start to reduce your supplement programme down to a level that will help to maintain your weight, shape and health. It should now include:

- a good multivitamin and mineral every day (from companies such as Solgar, the Natural Health Practice and Biocare)
- vitamin C 1,000mg every day
- Omega 3 fish oil capsules 1,000mg every day

But be prepared to add a vitamin B complex (with vitamins B5 and B6 adding up to 50mg – including what is already in the multivitamin and mineral) and Siberian ginseng (100mg) to boost your protection against stress hormones if you find yourself in a period of stress.

EXERCISE

You need to keep exercise in your life. Once you have got into the habit it is easy to keep it going. But you can ease off a bit if you like.

I would advise that you try to go to the gym once a week to do a combination of aerobics and weight-training. It is still useful to do the weight-training because as we get older we lose muscle which is why there is the tendency to gain weight with age. So the more muscle you can keep on, the more likely you are to stay at the weight you want.

Aim to get a little 'puffed out' for around thirty minutes, five times a week. But you don't have to don the lycra. This can just mean walking to the shops. The continued activity will be good for your weight and very good for your heart, immune system and digestion. And, as we have seen, it has also been proven effective in the prevention of Alzheimer's, so maintaining an exercise programme is good not only for your body but also your mind.

LIFESTYLE

If any area of your life starts to become a little stressful, just go back to Chapter 7 and see whether there are any strategies that you can employ that would help. Remember your breathing – however basic this sounds it really can make such a difference; by breathing correctly you are giving a strong message to your body that you are not under stress and can cope.

WHAT IF THE FAT AROUND THE MIDDLE STARTS TO CREEP BACK?

Whatever you do, don't despair. We all have our ups and downs. Just turn back to Chapter 10 and start again on the three-month four-prong attack (nutrition, supplements, exercise and lifestyle).

In my experience, because both you and your body now know the routine, the fat will actually come off quicker than before. This is because the last time you tried this plan you were giving your body a new message, telling it to burn fat rather than store it. This time, however, soon after you start back on the three-month programme, your body will get an 'Aha' moment and think, 'I've been here before'. The switch will take place much faster.

As American author Jim Rohn says, 'Take care of your body. It's the only place you have to live.' You not only want to look good and feel good but also to stay as free as you can from illness. By following the recommendations in this book and then keeping to a healthy way of eating most of the time, you will have put yourself on the path of good health.

And remember: eat well – keep fit – stay healthy!

RESOURCES

THE DR MARILYN GLENVILLE PHD CLINIC NATURAL HEALTHCARE FOR WOMEN

Feel free to call my clinic if you would like to have a consultation. Many of the tests mentioned in this book can be organised ahead of the consultation and the results can then be discussed either in person or by telephone.

Consultations

For an appointment at either of my clinics (in St John's Wood, London and Tunbridge Wells, Kent) and/or more information, please contact:

The Dr Marilyn Glenville Clinic, 14 St Johns Road, Tunbridge Wells, Kent TN4 9NP
Tel: 0870 5329244 Fax: 0870 5329255
Int. tel: +44 1 892 515905 Fax: +44 1 892 515914
Email: health@marilynglenville.com
Website: www.marilynglenville.com

Supplements and Tests

For more information or to order any of the supplements and tests mentioned in this go to:

The Natural Health Practice (NHP)
www.naturalhealthpractice.com/fataroundthemiddle
Tel: 0845 8800915 Int. tel: +44 1 892 507598

NHP is my supplier of choice and their range meets with all my recommendations – their supplements are all in the correct form and at the right dosage levels and they are made with the highest quality ingredients and free from all 'nasties' such as GMOs, sugar, preservatives. They are also non-allergenic.

On the NHP website 'Fat Around the Middle' page you will find everything that you need to follow the 'lose-your-belly' plan. This includes:

Supplements

'Lose your Belly' Nutri Plus
'Lose your Belly' Amino Plus

Tests

Adrenal stress test
Insulin resistance test
Yeast and parasite test
Food allergy test
Genetic tests

'Lose-your-belly' meal comparison

This is your own personal meal comparison to see how what you are eating now compares with what you should be eating.

'Slimmer You' photograph

Gives you a picture of what you will look like when you are slimmer – get one now!

REFERENCES

Chapter 1

1. Selye, H., 1978, *The Stress of Life*, New York, McGraw Hill.
2. Epel, E.S.S. *et al*, 2000, 'Stress and body shape: Stress-induced cortisol secretion is consistently greater among women with central fat', *Psychosomatic Medicine*, 62, 623–632.
3. Bjorntorp, P. and Rosmond, R., 2000, 'Neuroendrocrine abnormalities in visceral adiposity', *Int J Obes Relat Metab Disord*, 24, S2, S80–S85.

Chapter 2

1. Colditz, G.A. *et al*, 1995, 'Weight gain as a risk factor for clinical diabetes mellitus in women', *Ann Intern Med*, 122, 481–486 and Chan, J.M. *et al*, 1994, 'Obesity, fat distribution and weight gain as risk factors for clinical diabetes in men', *Diabetes Care*, 17, 961–969.
2. Hill, J.O. and Bessesen, D., 2003, Editorial, *Archives of Internal Medicine*, 4, 163, 395–397.
3. Pantanetti, P. *et al*, 2004, 'Adipose tissue as an endocrine organ? A review of recent data related to cardiovascular complications of endocrine dysfunctions', *Clin Exp Hypertens*, 26, 4, 387–398.
4. Konarzewska, J. and Wojclkowski, C., 'Risk of diabetes mellitus after pregnancy complicated by gestational diabetes mellitus (GDM)', *Ginekol Pol*, 75, 10, 754–759.
5. Chrousos, G.P., Torpy, D.J., Gold, P.W., 1998, 'Interactions between the hypothalamic-pituitary-adrenal axis and the female reproductive system: clinical implications', *Ann Intern Med*, 129:229–240.
6. Thomas, G. *et al*, 2005, 'Pre-natal anxiety predicts individual differences in cortisol in pre-adolescent children', *Biological Psychiatry*, 58, 211–217.
7. Kammerer, M. *et al*, 2002, 'Pregnant women become insensitive to cold stress', *BMC Pregnancy and Childbirth*, 1, 2, 8.
8. Scholl, T.O. and Chen, X., 2002, 'Insulin and the "thrifty" woman: the influence of insulin during pregnancy on gestational weight gain and postpartum weight retention', *Matern Child Health*, 6, 4, 255–261.
9. McTernan, P.G. *et al, 2002*, 'Glucocorticoid regulation of P450 aromatase activity in human adipose tissue: gender and site differences', *J Clin Endocr Metab*, 87, 1327–1336.
10. Isidori, A.M. *et al*, 1999, 'Leptin and androgen levels in male obesity', *J Clin Endocr and Metab*, 84, 3673–3680.

Chapter 3

1. Bjorntop, P. *et al*, 2000, 'Hypertension and the metabolic syndrome: closely related central origin', *Blood Pressure*, 9, 2–3, 71–82.
2. Whitmer, R.A. *et al*, 2005, 'Obesity in middle age and future risk of dementia: a 27-year longitudinal population-based study', *BMJ*, 330, 1360.
3. Giovannucci, E., 2005, 'The role of insulin resistance and hyperinsulinemia in cancer causation', *Current Medicinal Chemistry – Immunology, Endocrine and Metabolic Agents*, 5, 1, 53–60.
4. Chang, C.K. *et al*, 2003, 'Hyperinsulinemia and hyperglycaemia: possible risk factors of colorectal cancer among diabetic patients', *Diabetologia*, 46, 595–560.
5. Furberg, A.S. *et al*, 2004, 'Serum high-density lipoprotein cholesterol, metabolic profile and breast cancer risk', *J Nat Cancer Inst*, 96, 15, 1152–1160.
6. Berstein, L.M. *et al, 2004*, 'Insulin resistance, its consequences for the clinical course of the disease and possibilities of correction in endometrial cancer', *J Cancer Res Clin Oncol*, 130, 11, 687–693.
7. Augustin, L.S. *et al*, 2003, 'Dietary glycemic index, glycemic load and ovarian cancer risk: a case-controlled study in Italy', *Ann Oncol*, 14, 78–84.
8. Helgesson, O. *et al*, 2003, 'Self-reported stress levels predict subsequent breast cancer in a cohort of Swedish women', *Eur J Cancer Prev*, 12, 5, 377–381.

9. Lahmann, P.H. *et al*, 2003, 'A prospective study of adiposity and postmenopausal breast cancer risk: the Malmo diet and cancer study', *Int J Cancer*, 103, 246–252.
10. Huang, Z. *et al*, 1999, 'Waist circumference, waist hip ratio and risk of breast cancer in the Nurses' Health Study', *Am J Epidemol*, 150, 12, 1316–1324.
11. Silver, S.A. *et al*, 2005, 'Dietary carbohydrates and breast cancer risk: a prospective study of the roles of overall glycemic index and glycemic load', *Int J Cancer*, 114, 4, 653–658.
12. Solomon, C.G. *et al*, 2002, 'Menstrual cycle irregularity and risk for future cardiovascular disease', *J Clin Endocrinol Metabl*, 87, 5, 2013–2017.
13. Berga, S.L., 1995, 'Stress and Amenorrhoea', *Endocrinologist*, 5, 6, 416–421.
14. Nock, B., 1986, 'Norandrogenic regulation of progestin receptors: new findings, new questions, reproduction: a behavioural and neuroendocrine prospective', *Ann N Y Acad Sci*, 474, 415, 22.
15. Kiddy, D.S. *et al*, 1990, 'Differences in clinical and endocrine features between obese and non-obese subjects with polycystic ovary syndrome: an analysis of 263 consecutive cases', *Clinical Endocrinology*, 32, 213–220.
16. Epel, E.S. *et al*, 2004, 'Accelerated telomere shortening in response to life stress', *Proceedings of the National Academy of Sciences*, 101, 49, 17312–17315.
17. Ulrich, P. and Cerami, A., 2001, 'Protein glycation, diabetes and ageing', *Recent Prog Horm Res*, 56, 1–21.
18. Tamakoshi, K. *et al*, 2003, 'The metabolic syndrome is associated with elevated circulating C-reactive protein in healthy reference range, a systemic low-grade inflammatory state', *Int J Obesity*, 27, 443–449.
19. Cai, D. *et al*, 2005, 'Local and systemic insulin resistance resulting from hepatic activation of IKK-beta and NF-kappaB', *Nature Medicine*, 11, 2, 183–190.
20. Lee, A.L. *et al*, 2002, 'Stress and depression: possible links to neuron death in the hippocampus', *Bipolar Disord*, 4, 2, 117–128.

Chapter 4

1. Epel, E. *et al*, 2001, 'Stress may add bite to appetite in women: a laboratory study of stress-induced cortisol and eating behaviour', *Psychoneuroendocrinology*, 26, 1, 37–49.
2. Jenkins. D.J. *et al*, 1989, 'Nibbling versus gorging: metabolic advantages of increased meal frequency', *NEJM*, 321, 14, 929–934.
3. Khan, A. *et al*, 2003, 'Cinnamon improves glucose and lipids of people with Type 2 diabetes', *Diabetes Care*, 26, 12, 3215–3218.
4. Jenkins, D.J. *et al*, 1981, Glycemic index of foods: a physiological basis for carbohydrate exchange', *Am J Clin Nutr*, 34, 362–366.
5. Munro, J., 2005, 'Expressing the glycemic potency of foods', *Proc Nutr Soc*, 65, 115–122.
6. Brynes, A.E. *et al*, 2005, 'The beneficial effect of a diet with low glycaemic index on 24 hour glucose profiles in healthy young people assessed by continuous glucose monitoring', *Brit J Nutr*, 93, 2, 179–182.
7. Landin, K. *et al*, 1992, 'Guar gum improves insulin sensitivity, blood lipids, blood pressure, and fibrinolysis in healthy men', *Am J Clin Nutr*, 56, 1061–1065.
8. Leclere, C.J. *et al*, 1994, 'Amylose in legumes, peas, basmati, oat fibre significant for IR', *Am J Clin Nutr*, 59, 776S.
9. Romieu, I. *et al*, 2004, 'Carbohydrates and the risk of breast cancer among Mexican women', *Cancer Epidemiol Biomarkers Prev*, 13, 8, 1283–1289.
10. Pawlak, D.B. *et al*, 2004, 'Effects of dietary glycaemic index on adiposity, glucose homeostasis and plasma lipids in animals', *Lancet*, 364, 9436, 778–785.
11. Blundell, J.E. and Hill, A.J., 1986, 'Paradoxical effects of an intense sweetener (aspartame) on appetite', *The Lancet*, 1, 1092–1093.
12. Wurtman, R.J., 1983, 'Neurochemical changes following high dose aspartame with dietary carbohydrates', *New England Journal of Medicine*, 429–430.
13. Stegink, L.D. *et al*, 1989, 'Effect of repeated ingestion of aspartame-sweetened beverage on plasma amino acid, blood methanol and blood formate concentrations', *Metabolism*, 38, 4, 357–363.

14. Lipton, S.A. and Rosenberg, P.A., 1994, 'Excitatory amino acids as a final common pathway for neurologic disorders', *New England Journal of Medicine*, 300, 9, 613–622.
15. Layman, D.K., 2003, 'The role of leucine in weight loss diets and glucose homeostasis', *J Nutr*, 133, 1, 261S–267S.
16. Herbert, Y. and Thomas, R., 2000, 'Role of the insulin-like growth factor family in cancer development and progression', *J Nat Cancer Inst*, 92, 18, 1472–1489.
17. Larsson, S.C. *et al*, 2005, 'Milk, milk products and lactose intake and ovarian cancer risk: A meta-analysis of epidemiological studies', *Int J Cancer*, July 28 epub.
18. Willett, W.C., 1998, 'Dietary fat and obesity: an unconvincing relation', *Am J Clin Nutr*, 68, 6, 1149–1150.
19. Willett, W.C., 2002, 'Dietary fat plays a major role in obesity: no', *Obesity Reviews*, 3, 2, 59–68.
20. Stampfer, M.J. *et al*, 2000, 'Primary prevention of coronary heart disease in women through diet and lifestyle', *NEJM*, 343, 1, 16–22.
21. Emken, E.A. *et al*, *1992*, 'Comparison of dietary linolenic acid and linolenic metabolism in man: influence of dietary linoleic acid, Essential fatty acids and Eicosanoids'. *Invited papers from the Third International congress*, eds A. Sinclair and R. Gibson, American Oil Chemists Society, Illinois.
22. de Roos, N.M. *et al*, 2003, 'Trans fatty acids, HDL cholesterol and cardiovascular disease. Effects of dietary changes on vascular reactivity', *Eur J Med Res*, 8, 8, 355–357.
23. Mauger, J.F. *et al*, 2003, 'Effect of different forms of dietary hydrogenated fats on LDL particle size', *Am J Clin Nutr*, 78, 3, 370–375.
24. Stender, S. and Dyerberg, J., 2004, 'Influence of trans fatty acids on health', *Ann Nutri Metab*, 48, 2, 61–66.
25. Bastiaan, E. *et al*, 2003, 'Antecedent adrenaline attenuates the responsiveness to but not the release of counterregulatory hormones during subsequent hypoglycaemia', *J Clin Endocrin Metab*, 88, 11, 5462–5467.
26. Keijzers, G.B. *et al*, 2002, 'Caffeine can decrease insulin sensitivity in humans', *Diabetes Care*, 25, 2, 364–369.
27. Biagonni, I. and Davis, S.N., 2002, 'Caffeine: a cause of insulin resistance?', *Diabetes Care*, 25, 2, 399–400.
28. al'Absi, M. *et al*, 1998, 'Hypothalamic-pituitary-adrenocortical responses to psychological stress and caffeine in men at high and low risk for hypertension', *Psychosom Med*, 60, 4, 521–527.
29. Stafford, T., 2003, 'Psychology in the coffee shop', *Psychologist*, 16, 7, 358–359.
30. Dunwiddie, T.V. and Masino, S.A., 2001, 'The role and regulation of adenosine in the central nervous system', *Annual Review of Neuroscience*, 24, 31–55.
31. Garrett, B.E. and Griffiths, R.R., 1997, 'The role of dopamine in the behavioural effects of caffeine in animals and humans', *Pharmacology, Biochemistry and Behaviour*, 57, 533–541.
32. Komori, A. *et al*, 1993, 'Anticarcinogenic activity of green tea polyphenols', *Japan J Clin Oncol*, 23, 3, 186–190.
33. Imai, K. and Natachi, K., 1995, 'Cross sectional study of effects of drinking green tea on cardiovascular and liver diseases', *BMJ*, 310, 6981, 693–696.
34. Nagao, T. *et al*, 2005, 'Ingestion of tea rich in catechins leads to a reduction in body fat and malondialdehyde-modified LDL in men', *Am J Clin Nutr*, 81, 1, 122–129.
35. Bray, G.A. *et al*, 2004, 'Consumption of high-fructose corn syrup in beverages may play a role in the epidemic of obesity', *Am J Clin Nutr*, 79, 537–543.
36. Stampfer, M.J. *et al*, 2000, 'Primary prevention of coronary heart disease in women through diet and lifestyle', *NEJM*, 343, 1, 16–22.
37. Hu, F.B. *et al*, 2001, 'Diet, lifestyle and the risk of Type 2 diabetes mellitus in women', *NEJM*, 345, 790–797.

Chapter 5

1. Evans, G.W. and Pouchnik, D.J., 1993, 'Composition and biological activity of chromium-pyridine carbosylate complexes', *Journal of Inorganic Biochemistry*, 49, 177–187.
2. Anderson, R.A. *et al*, 1991, 'Supplemental chromium effects on glucose, insulin, glucagon and urinary chromium losses in subjects consuming controlled low-chromium diets', *Am J Clin Nutr*, 54, 909–916.

3. Evans, G.W. and Bowman, T.D., 1992, 'Chromium picolinate increases membrane fluidity and rate of insulin internalisation', *J Inorg Bio*, 46, 243–250.
4. No authors listed, 2004, 'A scientific review: the role of chromium in insulin resistance', *Diabetes Educ*, Suppl 2–14
5. Anderson, R.A., 1992, 'Chromium, glucose tolerance and diabetes', *Biological Trace Element Research*, 32, 19–24.
6. 'The Role of Chromium in Animal Nutrition, Committee on Animal Nutrition', *National Research Council*, 1997.
7. Bagchi, D. *et al*, 2002, 'Cytotoxicity and oxidative mechanisms of different forms of chromium', *Toxicology*, 180, 1, 5–22.
8. Ibid.
9. Walti, M.K. *et al*, 2003, 'Low plasma magnesium in Type 2 diabetes', *Swiss Med Weekly*, 133, 19–20, 289–292.
10. Takaya, J. *et al*, 2004, 'Intracellular magnesium and insulin resistance', *Magnes Res*, 17, 2, 126–136.
11. Kao, W.H. *et al*, 1999, 'Serum and dietary magnesium and the risk for Type 2 diabetes mellitus: the Atherosclerosis Risk in Communities Study', *Arch Intern Med*, 159, 18, 2151–2159.
12. Motoyama, T. *et al*, 1989, 'Oral magnesium supplementation in patients with essential hypertension', *Hypertension*, 13, 227–232.
13. Chen, M. D. *et al, 2000*, 'Zinc may be a mediator of leptin production in humans', *Life Sci*, 66, 22, 2143–2149.
14. Brandao-Neto, J. *et al*, 1990, 'Zinc acutely and temporarily inhibits adrenal cortisol secretion in humans. A preliminary report', *Biol Trace Elem Res*, 24, 1, 83–89.
15. Ford, E.S. *et al*, 2003, 'The metabolic syndrome and antioxidant concentrations: findings from the Third National Health and Nutrition Examination Survey', *Diabetes*, 52, 9, 2346–2352.
16. Chen, L. and Thacker, R., 1985, 'Effects of dietary vitamin E and high supplementation of vitamin C on plasma glucose and cholesterol levels', *Nutr Res*, 5, 527–534.
17. Johnston, C.S., 2005, 'Strategies for healthy weight loss: from vitamin C to the glycemic response', *J Am Coll Nutr*, 24, 158–165.
18. Enwonwu, C.O. *et al*, 1995, 'Effect of marginal ascorbic acid deficiency on saliva level of cortisol in the guinea pig', *Arch Oral Biol*, 40, 8, 737–742.
19. Peters, E.M. *et al*, 2001, 'Vitamin C supplementation attenuates the increases in circulating cortisol, adrenaline and anti-inflammatory polypeptides following ultramarathon running', *Int J Sports Med*, 22, 7, 537–543.
20. Wilburn, A.J. *et al*, 2004, 'The natural treatment of hypertension', *J Clin Hypertens*, 6, 5, 242–248.
21. National Diet and Nutrition Survey, 2003.
22. Koutsikos, D. *et al*, 1996, 'Oral glucose tolerance test after high dose i.v. biotin administration in normoglucemic hemodialysis patients', *Ren Fail*, 18, 131–133.
23. Setola, E. *et al*, 2004, 'Insulin resistance and endothelial function are improved after folate and vitamin B12 therapy in patients with metabolic syndrome: relationship between homocysteine levels and hyperinsulinemia', *Eur J Endocrinol*, 15, 4, 483–489.
24. Paolisso, G. *et al*, 1995, 'Chronic intake of pharmacological doses of vitamin E might be useful in the therapy of elderly patients with coronary heart disease', *Am J Clin Nutr*, 61, 4, 848–852.
25. Davi, G., 1999, 'In vivo formation of 8-iso-prostaglandin f2alpha and platelet activation in diabetes mellitus: effects of improved metabolic control and vitamin E supplementation', *Circulation*, 19, 2, 224–229.
26. Stephens, N.G., 1996, 'Randomised controlled trial of vitamin E in patients with coronary disease: Cambridge Heart Antioxidant Study (CHAOS)', *Lancet*, 347, 781–786.
27. Pryor, A., 2000, 'Vitamin E and heart disease: basic science to clinical intervention trial', *Free Radical Biology and Medicine*, 28, 141–164.
28. Holness, M.J. *et al*, 2003, 'Diabetogenic impact of long-chain omega-3 fatty acids on pancreatic beta-cell function and the regulation of endogenous glucose production', *Endocrinology*, 144, 9, 3958–68.
29. Wang, S. *et al*, 2001, 'Effects of chromium and fish oil on insulin resistance and leptin resistance in obese developing rats', *Wei Sheng Yan Jiu*, 30, 5, 284–286.
30. Van Gaal, L. *et al*, 1984, in: 'Folkers, K. Yamamura., eds: Biomedical and Clinical Aspects of Coenzyme Q10', *Elsevier Science Publ*, Amsterdam 4:369–373.

31. Shigeta, Y. *et al*, 1966, 'Effect of coenzyme Q10 treatment on blood sugar and ketone bodies of diabetics', *Journal of Vitaminology*, 12, 293–298.
32. Singh, R.B. *et al*, 1999, 'Effect of hydrosoluble coenzyme Q10 on blood pressures and insulin resistance in hypertensive patients with coronary artery disease', *J Hum Hypertens*, 13, 203–208.
33. Langsjoen, P.H. *et al*, 1990, 'A six year clinical study of therapy of cardiomyopathy with coenzyme Q10', *Int J Tissue React*, 12, 3, 169–171.
34. Konrad, T. *et al*, 1999, 'Alpha-lipoic acid treatment decreases serum lactate and pyruvate concentrations and improves glucose effectiveness in lean and obese patients with type 2 diabetes', *Diabetes Care*, 22, 2, 280–287.
35. El Midaoui, A. and de Champlain, J., 2002, 'Prevention of hypertension, insulin resistance and oxidative stress by alpha-lipoic acid', *Hypertension*, 39, 2, 303–307.
36. Fulghesu, A.M. *et al*, 2002, 'N-acetyl-cysteine treatment improves insulin sensitivity in women with polycystic ovary syndrome', *Fertil Steril*, 77, 6, 1128–1135.
37. Rogers, L.L. and Pelton, R.B., 1957, 'Glutamine in the treatment of alcoholism', *Q J Studies in Alcoholism*, 18, 581–587.
38. Neri, D.F. *et al*, 1995, 'The effects of tyrosine on cognitive performance during extended wakefulness', *Aviat Space Environ Med*, 66, 313–319.
39. Lin, J. *et al*, 2005, 'Green tea polyphenol epigallocatechin gallate inhibits adipogenesis and induces apoptosis in 3T3-L1 adipocytes', *Obes Res*, 13, 6, 982–990.
40. Yeh, G.Y. *et al*, 2003, 'Systematic review of herbs and dietary supplement for glycemic control in diabetes', *Diabetes Care*, 26, 4, 1277–1294.
41. Kim, D.H., 2003, 'Effects of ginseng saponin on hypothalamo-pituitary-adrenal axis in mice', *Neuroscience Letter*, 343, 62–66.
42. Spasov, A.A. *et al*, 2000, 'A double-blind, placebo-controlled pilot study of the stimulating and adaptogenic effect of Rhodiola rosea SHR-5 extract on the fatigue of students caused by stress during an examination period with a repeated low-dose regimen', *Phytomedicine*, 7, 2, 85–89.
43. Darbinvan, V. *et al*, 2000, 'Rhodiola rosea in stress induced fatigue – a double blind cross-over study of a standardized extract SHR-5 with a repeated low-dose regimen on the mental performance of healthy physicians during night duty', *Phytomedicine*, 7, 5, 365–371.

Chapter 6

1. Donnelly, J. *et al*, 2003, 'Effects of a 16 month randomized controlled exercise trial on body weight and composition in young, overweight men and women', *Arch Intern Med*, 163, 1343–1350.
2. Ryan, A.S. *et al*, 1996, 'Resistive training increases insulin action in postmenopausal women', *J Gerontol A Biol Sci Med Sci*, 51, M199–M205.
3. Mayer-Davis, E.J. *et al*, 1998, 'Intensity and amount of physical activity in relation to insulin sensitivity: the Insulin Resistance Atherosclerosis Study', *JAMA*, 279, 9, 669–674.
4. Randeva, H.S. *et al*, 2002, 'Exercise decreases plasma total homocysteine in overweight young women with polycystic ovary syndrome', *J Clin Endocrin Metab*, 87, 10, 4496–4501.
5. Miller, W.C. *et al*, 1997, 'A meta-analysis of the past 25 years of weight loss research using diet, exercise of diet plus exercise intervention', *Int J Obesity*, 21, 941–947.
6. Utter, A.C. *et al*, 1998, 'Influence of diet and/or exercise on body composition and cardiorespiratory fitness in obese women', *International Journal of Sport Nutrition*, 6, 213–222.
7. Miller, W.C. *et al*, 1997, 'A meta-analysis of the past 25 years of weight loss research using diet, exercise of diet plus exercise intervention', *Int J Obesity*, 21, 941–947.
8. Nelson, Miriam, 2000, *Strong Women Stay Young*, Bantam.
9. Ibid.
10. Aldred, H.E. *et al*, 1995, 'Influence of 12 weeks of training by brisk walking on postprandial lipemia and insulinemia in sedentary middle-aged women', *Metabolism*, 44, 390–397.
11. Grimm, J.J., 1999, 'Interaction of physical activity and diet: implications for insulin-glucose dynamics', *Public Health Nutr*, 2, 363–368.

Chapter 7

1. Touch Research Institute of the University of Miami School of Medicine, www.miami.edu/touch-research
2. Parati, G. and Steptoe, A., 2004, 'Stress reduction and blood pressure control in hypertension: a role for transcendental meditation?', *J Hypertens*, 22, 11, 2057–2060.
3. Brown, J., 1991, 'Staying Fit and Staying Well: Physical fitness as a moderator of life stress', *Journal of Personality and Social Psychology*, 60 (4) 555–561.
4. Grewen, K.M. *et al*, 2005, 'Effects of partner support on resting oxytocin, cortisol, norepinephrine, and blood pressure before and after warm partner contact', *Psychosomatic Medicine*, 67:531–538.
5. Kripke, D., Simons, R., Garfinkel, L. *et al*, 1979, 'Short and long sleep and sleeping pills. Is increased mortality associated?', *Arch Gen Psychiatry*, 36:103–116.
6. National Sleep Foundation, Sleep in America Poll, 2001–2002. Washington, DC: National Sleep Foundation.
7. Kern, W. *et al*, 1996, 'Changes in cortisol and growth hormone secretion during nocturnal sleep in the course of ageing', *Journal of Gerontology*, 51A, M3–9.
8. Spiegel, K. *et al*, 1999, 'Impact of sleep debt on metabolic and endocrine function', *Lancet*, 354, 1435–1439.
9. Sephton, S. and Spiegel, D., 2003, 'Circadian disruption in cancer: a neuroendocrine-immune pathway from stress to disease', *Brain Behav Immun*, 17, 5, 321–328.
10. Hasler, G. *et al*, 2004, 'The association between short sleep duration and obesity in young adults: a 13 year prospective study', *Sleep*, 27, 4, 661–666.
11. Spiegel, K. *et al*, 2004, 'Leptin levels are dependent on sleep duration: relationships with sympathovagal balance, carbohydrate regulation, cortisol and thyrotropin', *J Clin Endocrinol Metab*, 89, 11, 5762–5771.
12. Spiegel, K., Tasali, E., Penev, P. *et al*, 2004, 'Sleep curtailment in healthy young men is associated with decreased leptin levels: elevated ghrelin levels and increased hunger and appetite', *Ann Intern Med.* 141:846–850.
13. Taheri, S., Lin, L., Austin, D. *et al*, 2004, 'Short sleep duration is associated with reduced leptin, elevated ghrelin, and increased body mass index (BMI)', *Sleep*, 27: A146–A147.

Chapter 8

1. Loutan, L. and Lamotte, J.M., 1984, 'Seasonal variation in nutrition among a group of nomadic pastoralists in Niger', *Lancet*, 1, 945–947.
2. Bjorntorp, P., 2001, 'Do stress reactions cause abdominal obesity and comorbidities?', *Obes Rev*, 2, 2, 73–86.
3. Rosmond, R. *et al*, 2002, '5-HT2A receptor gene promoter polymorphism in relation to abdominal obesity and cortisol', *Obes Res*, 10, 7, 585–589.
4. Williams, P.T. *et al*, 2005, 'Concordant lipoprotein and weight responses to dietary fat change in identical twins with divergent exercise levels 1', *Am J Clin Nutr*, 82, 1, 181–187.

Chapter 9

1. Wallerius, S. *et al*, 2003, 'Rise in morning saliva cortisol is associated with abdominal obesity in men: a preliminary report', *J Endocrinol Invest*, 26, 7, 616–619.
2. Kronfol, Z. *et al*, 1997, 'Circadian immune measures in healthy volunteers: relationship to hypothalamic-pituitary-adrenal axis hormones and sympathetic neurotransmitters', *Psychom Med*, 59, 42–50.
3. Sephton, S.E. *et al*, 2000, 'Diurnal cortisol rhythm as a predictor of breast cancer survival', *J Nat Cancer Inst*, 92, 12, 994–1000.
4. Abercombie, H.C. *et al*, 2004, 'Flattened cortisol rhythms in metastatic breast cancer patients', *Psychoneuroendocrinology*, 29, 8, 1082–1092.
5. Yusaf, S. *et al*, 2004, 'Effect of potentially modifiable risk factors associated with myocardial infarction in 52 countries (the INTERHEART study): case-control study', *Lancet*, 364, 937–952.

INDEX